Chains of Autism

Yvonne Sanderson

Published by New Generation Publishing in 2024
Copyright © Yvonne Sanderson 2024

Brian Groom - Graphic Designer

ISBN: 978-1-83563-241-3

www.newgeneration-publishing.com

New Generation Publishing

Contents

Introduction to Chains of Autism

Having moved from Birmingham, England, in 1986 to start a new life with my partner in a small town of Staffordshire, life seemed to be working out. My daughter Kelly was born in 1987. I was enjoying being a mother and kept busy running our home. The social life I had previously enjoyed and the friends I had in Birmingham were no longer so important to me. Family life meant everything to me now.

My daughter was healthy, intelligent and making wonderful progress. Having another baby was, I thought, the natural way forward. My son Jonathan was born in 1989. I was happy and felt myself blessed to have two healthy children.

Four months after he was born, my life was going to change forever!

Jonathan contracted a virus and was hospitalised. As I watched the pain and distress he suffered, thoughts filled and raced through my head. When he came out of that terrible time, a mother's instinct told me that he would be affected.

The turmoil within my head continued. How did he contract the virus? Was it something I had done, or not done? I agonised that it must have been my fault.

I expressed my concerns with the doctors. I was told 'it is one of those things; he will get over it'. A comment was made that I was 'becoming over-protective'.

My son was discharged from hospital. There were no explanations about what could have caused his condition; no answers to my worries about how it may affect him.

I took my baby home, full of guilt, because I may have let him down and caused him to become ill.

Over the following twelve months, a health visitor came to the house to make regular checks on him. I raised questions about his lack of sleep, how he was not eating or drinking his milk, and how he was screaming constantly. He was getting worse.

My concerns were brushed off by the health visitor and I was accused again of being over protective and comparing him to his sister. I knew he had changed.

My partner found the situation difficult. He commented that I was spoiling Jonathan and not caring for our daughter as much as our son. Such comments were untrue and hurt me very deeply. I became very depressed by this, and thought myself a failure.

The pressure became too much and our relationship broke down. Now I was having to cope as a single parent too!

Over the next few years, Jonathan's behaviour became more challenging. The doctors sent him for a number of tests to try and find out what could be causing his problems, and we would wait for weeks in between each test for the results. The worry and stress consumed my every thought. Life was becoming unbearable, with no hope of it improving.

When the tests came back negative for anything life-threatening it was a huge relief for me, but it still was not giving me any reasons for his challenging behaviour, which was not 'normal' for a child approaching five years old.

The only solution the doctors could offer was medication to 'calm him down'. I refused to accept that this was the answer to his problems. I was finally told to look for a home to put him in and concentrate on my daughter. No way was I going to abandon my child.

The education authority did lots of assessments and reports and finally gave the diagnosis label of my son being autistic. They also gave me a list of residential schools that

I could send him away to, as the local special educational needs schools would not be able to manage his complex needs.

I did go to look at a number of the schools, but I knew after seeing them they would not benefit Jonathan. Hospital doctors and the education authority suggested

I 'send him away'. I came to the painful conclusion that I alone had to do all that was possible to enable my son to have the best life I could give him.

I informed the authorities I was opting out of the system. To my surprise, there was no opposition. I was now entirely on my own.

My journey takes place over the following twenty-five years, driven by the love of a mother believing in her son. I had to try and understand how he saw his world, to learn what being autistic was like for *him*.

Overcoming the obstacles and prejudice in society and determined to find out all I could how to help my son. Instead of focusing on what they can't do for their age, we should guide them towards things they can.

There are no milestones along the way to gauge progress as they age. They do not have the prospects of a career, travelling, setting up their own home, having a social life. As a mother, each day is filled with the fear of 'who will look after my child if I am no longer here?'

I wanted Jonathan to have a good quality of life, and be happy. The label 'autistic' was not going to prevent him having the opportunities to achieve all he could, within his capabilities. Autistic children need love, a great deal of patience and time from someone who believes in them to bring out the hidden talents that are within them.

Any single issue can take a long time to overcome or manage. I have broken my journey into five-year sections to help the reader understand an autistic child with complex issues.

It has been a very difficult journey with consequences that resulted in the breakdown of my health, and indeed almost took my life. Lack of money for healthy food, no sleep, and depressed about my son's future, I had to endure the unwanted stigma I felt having to rely on state benefits to survive.

My daughter was influenced to resent the attention her brother needed. That resentment from her has grown over the years. Our relationship deteriorated to the point of my daughter's complete ostracisation of me. It saddens me to have to accept there is little prospect of that changing in the future. She is making her own choices about her life, which is what any mother wants for her children. Unfortunately, her brother cannot do that. He needs help and support.

To see how Jonathan is today, and the achievements he has made, I know it was all worthwhile.

This is the story of our journey. I hope it will help and inspire others who are in a similar position, and those who can do something to understand.

Names and places have been changed to protect identities.

Chapter One - The First Five Years

When the doctors at the hospital said I could take Jonathan home, as he had finished his treatment, I felt frightened deep down. Worried I might not be able to cope with caring for him as he was.

I had watched my baby's struggle to survive. I felt helpless to do anything. The nurses and doctors were monitoring his health. At home, I would be on my own.

With no answers to allay my concerns and fears, it was just expected that I would settle back into normal life.

My daughter was happy that we were back home and that she could see her brother again. My partner was eager to return to work after having had time off to look after Kelly. We had no extended family to help out and hadn't made any new friends in the area.

I tried to get into a family routine again and making sure Kelly didn't feel left out with me caring for a new baby. Her father was now at work, his attention she had to herself while Jonathan was in hospital.

It wasn't long before she commented that Jonathan was always crying and I had to pick him up a lot. She lost interest in her baby brother. She would tell this to her father on his return from work.

I tried to explain that he wasn't sleeping much, not feeding very well, and seemed to be in pain, for reasons I couldn't understand.

The health visitor was not overly concerned when I raised these issues. She seemed casually to dismiss them, putting it down to my 'not getting into a routine', or 'spoiling him by picking him up all the time'. What caring mother would not pick up her constantly screaming child to comfort them?

To my surprise, my partner agreed with the health visitor's comments. (These comments hurt me very deeply.) With no support, I was increasingly tired and depressed. I was scared to share my fears that the virus had damaged Jonathan. This fear was constantly on my mind.

My partner started complaining about his lack of sleep and having to get up for work. I decided to stay downstairs with Jonathan at night so I could try and keep him quiet, to let my daughter and partner get some sleep.

The stress was becoming unbearable for all. Family life had become a nightmare. I *knew* my son had changed. I felt guilty about the whole situation, with nowhere to turn to for help.

The following twelve months were a struggle trying to care for Jonathan. He was still not in any routine, his behaviour was getting worse, and the demands on me were affecting my mental and physical health.

Fear and worry about Jonathan's development had taken over my every thought, day and night. I wasn't comparing him with my daughter, who was progressing well under the circumstances. I put a great deal of effort into spending what time I could during the day with her. I recognise that this wasn't enough. Her father's attention made up for that when he was at home. I saw she was happy about that.

Jonathan was approaching two years old, and not developing as a child of that age is expected to.

Trips out to the park, so Kelly could play and meet other children, would always end in us having to leave after a short while because Jonathan would scream and cry and thrash about in his pushchair. He refused to get out of his pushchair to play. His distress continued until I took him from the environment. Other parents would make comments like 'why can't she control him?' and Kelly would get upset at having to leave the park. She resented it. This made me feel as though I didn't want to leave the house at all!

Shopping was a similar ordeal. One supermarket opened at 7 a.m. and I used to try and do the shopping when it was quietest.

All too often something would upset Jonathan and cause him to scream and thrash about; it could be a person talking loudly, a child shouting or crying; any sudden noise, or a shop assistant making harsh comments. As Jonathan started to become upset, I knew I had to abandon the visit immediately and the shopping until another day. I had to explain several times to managers about the problems I was experiencing with Jonathan, and coming early in the mornings was the only way for me to shop.

Again, I felt sorry for Kelly that she had to put up with these inconveniences. I felt really disappointed for her, but I couldn't do anything other than take Jonathan home.

It was the same when I had to go to a bank or post office, which didn't open early, and there were usually lots of people around. Every time I was out with my children, I felt people were judging me!

This feeling was making me more depressed. Jonathan's behaviour was not 'normal', and I couldn't understand why.

The relationship with my partner broke down. We were under a great deal of stress. We could not agree about the fears I had for Jonathan, that the virus had affected him and was the cause of his issues, not me spoiling him.

I was now having to cope as a single parent, I was consumed with guilt and scared for my son's future.

He was not attempting to talk. Not a single word! Not even that word I longed to hear: mommy.

He had no sense of day or night. No interaction with his sister. He just wanted to be away from her.

The only thing that seemed to calm him was playing alone with his toy trains.

Jonathan was developing a dislike for wearing clothes. Getting him dressed to go out was a real challenge. He just wanted to wear his pyjamas.

If it was cold outside, he still would not want to wear his hat, coat, gloves and would try his best to pull them off.

If he saw snow in the garden, he would want to play out in it, whatever time of day or night it was. I used to dread the winter months. I knew the problems that would have to be dealt with when Jonathan wanted to play out. I tried to distract him from looking out of the window at night if there was snow. I would keep playing his favourite *Thomas the Tank Engine* videos. This didn't always work! One very cold night, he noticed snow outside and wanted to go and play. I couldn't distract him or stop him becoming distressed. My daughter was asleep, as it was 2 a.m.! I had to take him out. He would not put on a coat or hat or gloves. It was a struggle to get his shoes on. He wanted to go out in his pyjamas.

This occasion brought me to the point of desperation. I cried out loud, 'I can't go on like this anymore!'

I looked at Jonathan: he was not even aware of how cold he was. (That struck me as very strange!) I was freezing cold. I just picked him up and took him back into the house, got him changed and sat with him to watch his videos until Kelly woke up. I was exhausted from crying, and was having thoughts like 'how much more can I cope with?'

As time went on, Jonathan was having more problems. He did not have much of an appetite and refused to eat anything apart from white bread and pasta. He was reluctant to wear clothes. He didn't like wet nappies against his skin and would try to pull them off. This gave me the idea to try potty training him. I would take him to his potty at regular times during the day and night (because he didn't sleep). It was some months later he had learnt to use the potty then toilet. This showed me that although he couldn't ask to go, he could be taught. If he could be taught that, he must be capable of doing more.

I discussed his development issues with the health visitor (who was most surprised that he had been toilet trained), and they agreed to refer him to his doctor to arrange some tests.

His behaviour was worse and not 'normal' for a child approaching three years old.

I felt a huge relief that at last someone was listening to me, and there might be some answers to his condition.

The following year was taken up by a series of testing that seemed to have no end. They were very upsetting for my son and me. They told me they would be testing for a number of conditions I had never heard of, such as Fragile X and Muscular Dystrophy. I would worry myself, asking, 'how will I cope if it is this, or that?'

In between each test and waiting for the results seemed to be an eternity. As each test came back negative for anything life threatening. My mind was in turmoil. I had convinced myself one of these tests would show something to explain Jonathan's behaviour.

When the doctors could not provide me with an answer, they suggested the education authority may be able to help.

Over the following months lots of assessments were done with Jonathan at home, focusing on what he could not do. The education authority suggested I send him to a special educational needs nursery where further assessments could be carried out, to help them decide what school he should go to.

I felt that my son's future was being decided by people who didn't know him, and by assessments of what he couldn't do for his age, now four and a half.

I was very angry inside. I knew I had to go along with them to try and understand why Jonathan was behaving the way he was. He would go to the special educational needs nursery two mornings a week. It used to break my heart to take him and have to leave him, but I had no choice.

My daughter was at school, and it gave me a chance to visit the library and research anything I could on child development. This took my mind off worrying about Jonathan, and the time went by quickly. When I went to pick him up, I was filled with dread and anger each time I went into the nursery. I couldn't see how it was helping my son. He was always crying and distressed; as I picked him up, I wondered what assessments were they doing.

Finally, the reports had been completed. The diagnosis label they had given my son was autistic. I didn't know anything about it.

The education authority informed me that the local special educational needs school would not be able to manage his complex needs, as he required one-to-one attention which they could not offer at that time or in the foreseeable future.

They gave me a list of residential schools to look at, and I could choose one that he would go away to.

The reports went to the paediatrician at the hospital. At the final appointment the paediatrician made a remark to me: 'find a home to put him in, and concentrate on your daughter.' I was very hurt by this. The medical authorities had now given up on my son and considered him to have no future. I was never going to give up on him.

I did visit a few of the schools, and I knew I could not put my son into a place like those I saw.

After a great deal of thought, I came to the decision I would do all within my power to help my son.

I was going to opt out of the system.

After informing the education authority of my decision. To my surprise, there was no opposition. They informed me that I must put it in writing for them to close Jonathan's file and shred it. This would take a couple of weeks, and Jonathan would complete his last few sessions at nursery.

I took the opportunity to research in the library to find anything I could on autism. There was not much that was helpful. What I did find was two addresses of clinics that dealt with child development. I wrote down the information. I felt it was a start; a lead.

I didn't consider that one was in Israel, and the other in America.

I sent a letter to each clinic explaining how Jonathan was behaving, and to ask if there was any information, they could give me. I was hoping deep down they would get in touch with me, but worried too, because I had no chance of ever visiting either clinic. I had no money, was living on state benefits, but sending a letter gave me a little hope of finding something out about how to help my son, who was approaching five years old and had no hope of a future that any mother has for her child.

The nursery sessions had finished; I felt a great relief, because Jonathan had not benefited from being there. He had been labelled for the rest of his life as autistic.

Within a few weeks of me sending the letters to the clinics I had a reply from both of them. The first was from Israel, explaining they didn't see children until they were eight years old. They also listed some dates and places for lectures held in the United Kingdom by a professor from the clinic. I was disappointed, but I knew I couldn't wait until Jonathan was eight. Soon after I got a reply from the clinic in America, who gave me details of a clinic they work with closely in the United Kingdom, and the address was in Somerset.

I couldn't believe what I was reading! This was somewhere which I could travel to. They might be able to help Jonathan.

I phoned them and started the process. I was overwhelmed with emotion that I had found somewhere to help us.

It didn't really frighten me when I found out that the clinic was private and I would have to pay. All I could focus on was they felt that the clinic would be able to offer guidance.

After being sent all the paperwork to complete before visiting, which I filled out as soon as possible, I began thinking about the money. How was I going to pay for the first appointment? There wasn't enough money to live on and pay bills. I was working out where I could cut back further on things like food and heating to try to get the first payment.

I had to go to the clinic. It was my only hope to help Jonathan. I couldn't go on living as we were. My mental and physical health would not cope with the tremendous stress and fear that took over me every minute of every day.

I decided to seek a bank loan. I was honest about the whole situation and set plans on how I would pay the money back, if I could be trusted with the loan to cover the costs of the appointment. It was a very difficult request but I needed the money and would make sure it was paid back.

At last, one accepted my application! For this I will always be humbly grateful. I was trusted and believed in.

Chapter Two Five to Ten Years Old

The appointment came through to go to the clinic. It would mean Jonathan and I being there for a week. I was very worried and anxious because I had no idea how we would get through it and didn't really know what to expect. I had no choice, as there was nowhere else that could help my son. I arranged for my daughter to be looked after by her father.

The first morning at the clinic was meeting with the therapists and giving them information on Jonathan's behaviour. They could see how he was becoming more distressed and started running about, banging on the door of the room we were in, to get out. He was screaming and pulling at my arm to take him out of the situation. I was getting upset watching him, and questioned myself, 'why have I come here?'

The medical doctor and therapists kept reassuring me not to worry about how he was behaving. That was what I was there for. They needed to see Jonathan as he was, so they could find out about his problems.

After a very stressful morning, it was time for a lunch break in the dining room. There were a variety of foods but Jonathan would not eat anything. He wanted white bread or pasta, which they didn't have. I tried to persuade him to try something else, but he refused. This was being observed and noted by the therapist.

The afternoon was spent in a playroom. It had lots of different toys and colourful objects to help Jonathan try a number of activities. He wasn't very happy or cooperative as they did not have any toy trains to play with.

He was observed on things like how he picked up items, which hand he used, and how he tried to throw a ball. There were activities to see if he could pick up small things with his fingers.

I began to realise he had problems that I hadn't noticed before, because life was so stressful. Now, it was being shown to me.

The clinic informed me that Jonathan would be videoed during the visit to help the therapists put together a programme at the end of the week of tasks that could help him over time with his issues. Also, during the week, I would attend a one-day lecture to help me understand more about the programme and the brain; how our senses can affect our lives if they are imbalanced.

I was worried about leaving Jonathan with the therapists while I went to the lecture, but they reassured me he would be doing other fun activities. During the lecture a member of staff would come in to let me know he was alright and give me some tablets for my constant headaches.

I tried to settle down and understand what was being said. The lecture was given by the founder of the clinic. He had set it up some years before to help his disabled daughter. As he could not find anywhere in this country to help, he went to America, where he found a clinic that offered alternative therapies to stimulate the brain and senses that were non-invasive and did not use medication. After he came back from America, he sold his house to set up the clinic.

The information on the brain and senses was very interesting, and I thought to myself, 'we are parents here trying to help our children. Doctors should be learning this. I felt angry that my son's paediatrician never mentioned any of this!'

The founder was trying to give us as much information as possible on the programme that we would take home to work on. He understood the desperation we parents felt. He pointed out that we were at the end of the road and it was true, because he had been there too!

By the end of the week, Jonathan and I were exhausted. Neither of us had eaten or slept much. I was worried about the outcome; whether the clinic could really offer any help.

On the last day I went into the room to meet with the therapists, who had put together a programme. To enable me to take it all in, Jonathan was looked after by a member of staff.

The therapists explained that Jonathan's sense of smell was extremely acute. He could smell different people and this was why he was reacting to certain environments and people near him.

His hearing was very sensitive too and everything sounded loud to him, which would cause him pain and make him scream.

His nervous system was also affected. Different materials, like his clothes, felt like glass against his skin. It affected his senses to feel anything hot or cold.

They gave me examples to try so I could understand how Jonathan felt.

The strong smell made me feel sick, the loud noises they demonstrated made me realise how it would give him headaches, but he couldn't tell me, only scream and cry.

His clothes feeling like glass helped me to understand why he kept pulling them off. His taste buds could only tolerate bland foods, like white bread or pasta.

He also had coordination problems. Even though he could walk, he could not kick a ball, throw or catch one. He could not pick up small things because of his dexterity problems.

All the observations were videoed too, and they could show me the difficulties he had doing the activities.

I was astounded by how much had been found out about Jonathan. Most of all, it made sense to me.

The team of therapists did make a statement that shocked me. They said if I didn't try to do something now. Jonathan would be institutionalised by the age of ten or eleven years old, because he could not live in the 'real world'.

Two therapists would come to the house after three months to see if there was any progress. The cost was included in the assessment. They explained that the programme may help Jonathan over time, but there was no guarantee. I accepted that but was glad I had something to try.

Relieved to be going home after a very stressful but informative week, the founder of the clinic came to say bye to us. I will always remember what he said: 'Don't ever put limitations on him.'

I didn't fully understand what he meant then, but over time I began to realise it.

He also suggested when we get home to put the programme away for a week, settle down and grasp everything I had learnt, then work out a plan on how to implement it into our daily lives.

I wanted to start on the programme straight away. I looked at the list of different things that needed to be done every day. I decided to start with the cassette tape that they had given me. It was of different sounds and frequencies that lasted three minutes but needed to be played twelve times a day, with intervals of 20-30 minutes. I felt it was a start, and something I could understand might help him calm down in time.

At first, he didn't take any notice of the sounds playing. It wasn't unpleasant to listen to, just 'different.' When Jonathan was watching his *Thomas the Tank Engine* videos, I would turn the tape up a little and watch his reaction. Over the first few days, I played the tape as much as I could. When I had completed the twelve times, I decided to put it on during the night, hoping it would make a difference sooner if he listened to it more. After a week or so, it was becoming part of Jonathan's routine. My daughter would complain that she didn't like it on, asking why I had to play it so much. I explained it was to help Jonathan's sensitive hearing, and it needed to be played as much as possible.

The next part of the programme was to introduce different smells. Aromatherapy oils were suggested; I could either burn them in a diffuser around the house, or just ask him to smell different ones throughout the day. The oils were expensive so I decided to buy one each week. As the weather was getting colder, being November, I could keep the windows closed and the different smells would stay in the room. Some oils Jonathan liked better than others, and I was beginning to understand how this exercise was helping him.

Another part of the programme aimed to desensitise his hearing over time by getting him to experience a variety of sounds without any warning. For example, I would bang two saucepan lids loudly, or drop them on the floor or in the sink and observe his reactions to the sounds.

I knew he liked wearing his pyjamas because they were a soft material. So, I had to make sure all of his clothes were made of a material he could tolerate. I was becoming more aware of the things that caused him distress, even if he was unable to communicate why.

The part of the programme that aimed to help with his coordination problems involved being outside in the garden. It would be throwing, catching or kicking a ball and running a little. Having to concentrate on each task was helping me to realise that Jonathan had many issues that needed working on, and I knew it was going to take a long time.

As time went on, I was becoming more engrossed in completing each part of the programme and extending it to night-time too.

My daughter's objections to the time and attention her brother was being given did make me feel guilty about not having enough time with her. I tried to explain to her that Jonathan can't be like her because of all his problems and the different things I was doing with him would help to calm him down and in time be able to play with her.

She pointed out to me that Christmas was coming, and she did not want him to spoil it again for her. I hadn't realised the Christmas season was so close. I had been so involved in the programme and the time was going by so fast. I had not been able to visit the local toy shop since before going to the clinic. They had a saving scheme which enabled me to save what I could afford throughout the year to buy Christmas toys for the children. I didn't have any more money saved. All I had left was enough to buy aromatherapy oils that Jonathan needed for his programme. I knew the amount already paid to the shop would only be enough to buy Kelly a few of the toys she had asked for.

Jonathan did not enjoy Christmas, because he didn't understand it as Kelly, or any child without autism did. He would open his presents with no reaction of joy. He could not cope with the decorations or Christmas tree, or Christmas songs. Everything that I tried to help both children feel part of the season seemed to distress Jonathan. He would want the Christmas tree taken down after he had opened his presents. To him it was 'over' and he wanted it all put away. I had to struggle each year with him, pulling at the tree to take it down, which used to upset Kelly very much. Some years it came down on Christmas Day, other years I managed to get through until the next morning.

This year I was feeling more anxious and worried about what will happen. My daughter was determined Jonathan was not going to spoil it again for her; which meant however distressed he became about the Christmas tree it was not coming down! I knew I had to try and make it a happy day for her. I decided to get Jonathan one toy train and use the rest of the money for Kelly's gifts. Jonathan would not understand and would be pleased with his train.

Kelly would feel that she had got more than her brother, and that would make her feel 'special'.

I was worrying about the visit just after Christmas from the therapists at the clinic. I knew Jonathan did not like people coming to the house.

Christmas Day came and it went by without too much stress. Kelly liked her presents, and Jonathan his train. When he wanted the Christmas tree taken down, I managed to distract him by putting on the sound tape several times and played his *Thomas the Tank Engine* videos. Kelly had to take it in turns with him to watch her programmes, which she resented, but at least the decorations stayed up. I accept how difficult it must have been for my daughter, and I felt deep down she was blaming and resenting me.

I carried on throughout the day with the aromatherapy oils and played catch with a ball, which Kelly could get involved with for a short time. I began to realise that Jonathan was accepting parts of the programme into his daily life.

With Christmas over and the decorations put away, I could focus on Jonathan's programme. I could not see any great progress, but I noticed the little things, like being able to cope with the tree and decorations up until the next day. He let his sister watch her television programmes when it was her turn. I encouraged him to let me play with him and his toy trains. It was only for a short time, but to me it was progress. Although he was still not talking, he was interacting through his trains.

January came, and the day of the visit from the therapists at the clinic. There were two of them. At 9 a.m. they knocked on the door. To my surprise Jonathan came to the door with me and recognised the two people from the clinic. He was calm and did not get stressed as I expected. They were talking to him about his trains and he did not scream or run about. We went through a few of the exercises on the programme, and he was cooperating!

They were very pleased at his progress in such a short time, and suggested we go back to the clinic in six to twelve months for an update, but for only two days.

I explained about the loan I had for the first visit, and I would need to pay that off before I could think about another appointment.

The therapists gave me hope that the programme was helping Jonathan, and it was up to me how long I carried on with it.

When their visit finished, I began to think about what was said on the progress Jonathan was making. I hadn't really noticed until the therapists came to the house. I felt the three months of trying the programme had helped more than I realised. I had to continue with it as part of our daily lives.

Even though Jonathan was still not talking, he was a little calmer in his behaviour.

The coordination exercises that needed to be done in the garden were becoming a problem. The weather didn't seem to put him off trying, it was hearing a dog bark in another garden. He would run into the house. We had a high fence around the garden, and a dog could not have got in. It would cause him anguish and distress. I knew we couldn't carry on outside. If a bird flew over him near him, he would be frightened and again, that would end the exercises. As would flies or butterflies flying about him. All caused him to react with fear.

I knew he was starting to enjoy the ball games and running and jumping exercises. So, I decided to ask at our local leisure centre about hiring a hall for a few hours a week to help him continue with the programme. The manager was very helpful and kindly let us use the hall and soft play equipment at a low cost. This would also mean Jonathan was going out of the house to a different environment. It would take time to introduce this to him. After a while of going to the leisure centre and showing him the hall with different things to have fun with, he began to kick a ball and run around freely with me. I could see how I could build on this activity each time we came.

It did feel lonely at times, just the two of us. Jonathan did have the understanding and was calmer being without other children around him, because he wouldn't be able to cope with the noise. I had to keep telling myself why I was doing it this way.

It took many months for him to improve his coordination skills. It may have been just kicking a ball back and forth to me or catching a ball and throwing it to me. Whenever there was a moment like that, it gave me hope that he was progressing, and that kept me going. I knew his coordination problems would have to be worked on for many years to come, as with the other sensory issues he had.

For the little progress Jonathan was making over time, which kept me going for another day, life was becoming more difficult. Money was very scarce and I was finding it harder to cope with everything. I had to cut back on bills and was behind in payments, living with the hope that as soon as the loan was paid off things would improve.

To add to my problems, I found out that Kelly was having difficulties at school. One day her head teacher called me in to discuss the situation. I explained the circumstances around having Jonathan at home. He seemed to know quite a lot about what was going on at home. Kelly had commented on 'how she can't get any sleep; and her mother's time is spent sorting him out.' There were other issues about how she felt left out.

The head teacher was understanding, but stated he felt she wasn't cooperating in class and was finding it difficult to mix with the other children. I asked if she was behind with her work. The answer was no, which I was relieved about. Kelly had said it was all too easy.

Having listened to the head teacher I felt very guilty that I hadn't realised Kelly was having problems sooner. I was so engrossed every day trying to do the programme and taking Kelly to and from school. I had thought that part of life was working out.

I asked the head teacher what would be the best solution to this problem. His answer was to take her out of school. I was shocked and hurt. It wasn't her fault about how we were living. I was trying my best to give her time. She was a very intelligent child, and yet her school didn't want her there.

I was angry and upset. Trying not to show my feelings in front of the head teacher. I asked about the paperwork that needed to be done and left the school. I did not know how I would cope with two children that had different needs to teach at home.

The education authority informed me they would send an inspector out once a year to check on Kelly's progress. There was no mention of Jonathan.

I told the children's father about the school and that Kelly would be learning at home. He said he would help with her education.

The first few months of not having to take Kelly to and from school was in a way taking a little stress off me, and the demands I had to deal with daily. If Jonathan had woken Kelly during the night, I knew she could catch up with her sleep later, without worrying about being tired for school.

It took me a while to try to work out a routine to make sure Jonathan's sensory exercises were done, and Kelly was doing her work. It was difficult for us all. I hadn't slept for one complete night for almost six years; just an hour here and there if Jonathan slept. I felt I was always exhausted, and getting more depressed, with the added pressure of making sure Kelly did her work. She was ahead in intelligence for her eight years, and it worried me about how to set the level of work. I decided to get some books from the library on the Key Stages she currently needed to work on and some more advanced ones too.

At first Kelly would cooperate with working at home knowing a great deal of the day was taken up with Jonathan's programme and managing his behaviour. After a while, she decided to spend more time at her father's house to do the work with him, which meant staying overnight more often than I liked her doing. She began to see it as a way of getting away from Jonathan and me. As I felt responsible for her having to come out of school, I couldn't stand in her way of being with her father, who was helping with her education. I had no choice. Jonathan needed one-to-one care twenty-four hours a day, and I had 'chosen' to take him out of the system.

I did involve Kelly as much as I could with Jonathan's programme. When we went to the leisure centre to do ball games she enjoyed joining in for a while, and I could see Jonathan was starting to get used to her being with us, and didn't become stressed at taking turns to throw, or pass a ball to each other.

I was aware of Kelly not being with other children and found a drama and dancing group for her to go to. It also made me realise Jonathan was on his own. He had me but was not mixing with other children. Over time, I asked Kelly if she wanted to bring a friend home from time to time from her groups. My hope was not only to help her social skills, but to see how Jonathan coped with having other children in the house.

As Kelly thought about the idea and asked the friends she knew from her groups, I spoke to the parents about dates and times. I felt the need to explain Jonathan's behaviour issues – to get their reaction, and to see if they felt comfortable with their child coming to our house. Sadly, it did result in one or two of Kelly's friends not being allowed to come. The ones that did come were friendly towards Jonathan and wanted to play with him and his toys. I was really pleased he was being accepted by other children! What I also observed was that Kelly didn't like her friends playing with her brother. They were 'her' friends. As they inevitably fell out between themselves, Kelly decided that she wasn't going to have her friends at the house.

I began to understand the effect our family circumstances were having not only on myself and Jonathan, but my daughter too. I tried my best to help her socialise, and I knew she was resenting Jonathan more. He wasn't talking, didn't play with her, kept disturbing her nights; making every aspect of her life difficult. Most of all, I felt she was blaming me.

It was during an argument she was having with me one day about Jonathan getting his own way over the television. She shouted at me and Jonathan, 'He's just stupid, and he can't even talk or read!'

I could not believe what she was saying. I knew she was angry but I felt very hurt that she really meant what she was saying about her brother.

I just said angrily back, 'He's not stupid, he can't help the way he is. That is why I am doing the different things to try and help him improve, and maybe one day talk!'

She chose to spend more time with her father over the following weeks.

I was starting to wonder what I was doing to my children. My daughter was choosing not to be with me. She couldn't understand about her brother's condition, nor could I expect a child of eight years old to. I was struggling to come to terms with it all. My son had no future. He couldn't live in the 'real world' unless his sensory issues were desensitised somehow. He was not able to communicate through speech. His appetite was restricted to bland foods, and he was reluctant to try different foods. He would not sleep for any longer than one or two hours at a time. He had no sense of time of the day or night. I was on my own, out of the system with no support.

My biggest concern was not knowing who would look after him if anything happened to me. No one would be able to control his behaviour and he would, as the clinic pointed out to me, be institutionalised. I began to wonder what the point of it all was. The medical professionals and education authority had given up on my son. His father did not see the point of the programme I was working on from the clinic. My daughter was having less to do with me and Jonathan. It all seemed like a nightmare! The only thought of any hope I had to cling onto was the information the clinic had given me after observing Jonathan and showing me on video. It all made sense to me. Deep down I knew if I could just carry on working on the issues he had, one day he might improve. I had to carry on doing what I could to help Jonathan, hoping my daughter would be able to understand the reasons when she was older. She would grow up, get a job, have her own life. My son would not be able to do that, however much I worked on his sensory and coordination problems. As his mother, I was the only person who really loved and cared enough about him, and wanted to do all I could to give him some quality of life. I was trying to understand how he saw the world and what upset him about everyday life. Nothing else mattered to me. I loved my daughter and did all I possibly could but I had to accept the consequences of the decisions I'd made, and how I let her down, because of the drive to help Jonathan improve enough to not be institutionalised.

The thought filled me with dread, but it made me more determined than ever to do everything I could to prevent it happening.

The year following the visit to the clinic was taken up with working on Jonathan's sensory and coordination issues. I decided to start training him to stay in his own bedroom at night. We had spent so long living downstairs; he hardly used his own room. It would also get him into the routine of going to bed at night and not watching videos. I explained to Kelly what I was doing, that he would probably make a noise to start with, but I had to try.

It was extremely difficult at the beginning; turning off his videos and going into his own room. I played the sound tape to try and keep him calm. He did not want to stay in his room. I tried to distract him with looking at his train books and sitting on his bed, hoping he would settle. I set myself a time limit to aim for at keeping him in his room. Fifteen minutes, before he became loud and distressed, until I let him go downstairs. This went on for many months, building up from fifteen minutes up to an hour, then eventually three or four hours. It was very exhausting and stressful, because I felt I was being cruel by not letting him go downstairs. I knew if he was ever going to live a 'normal' life, he must learn to live in a routine. Sometimes he would fall asleep for a short while and so did I, and I felt as though progress was being made, however small.

His speech was still not improving, but his behaviour was becoming more manageable. I had stuck in my mind, 'I must keep trying everything to help him before he reaches ten years old, when he may have to be institutionalised if he hasn't improved.' This thought tormented me every waking minute. Through fear of that happening, I would push myself harder each day to make sure he was completing all of the exercises. Taking into account his lack of appetite, I would try him with a new taste of food to encourage him away from white bread and pasta. I would put some peas on the plate with his pasta or give him some brown bread. All my attempts were refused, but I was determined to keep trying until I found something he would eat along with his usual foods.

At the supermarket, I saw children's cereal boxes with colourful pictures on them. I showed them to Jonathan, who was not interested, but I still bought a few boxes to encourage him with. As I was buying different items of food each week to introduce to him, these extra things were adding more to the food bill. I decided to cut back on my food to allow me to buy the other foods for Jonathan, even though I knew it would be wasted unless Kelly chose to eat them. I understood Jonathan's taste was for bland foods, but I was hoping that would change over time.

With my life taken up caring for Jonathan and trying to work on all of his issues we were very much confined to the home except for shopping, the leisure centre, or the bank. Life had no joy or happiness. Nothing to look forward to. It was just stress and trying to limit it on a daily basis.

Jonathan, who was approaching seven years old, was not able to communicate verbally. He did not interact with his sister and preferred to play alone with his toy trains. He could not dress or wash himself without help and needed me to stay with him all of the time when it was bedtime. His lack of sleep meant he would want to go downstairs to play with his trains at 3 or 4 a.m., which resulted in complaints from my neighbour.

He would make noises when playing, crashing the trains together or throwing them off the table. As much as I tried to keep him calm, the noises did sound loud. On one particular occasion, I had a knock at the door at 7 a.m. It was a policeman. He said a neighbour had complained about the noise every night into the early hours of the morning. I asked him to come and see for himself what the situation was. I explained Jonathan's behaviour, how I was trying to keep him calm whilst my daughter got some sleep. I did my best to keep the noise down and didn't feel the noise would upset the neighbours.

I explained that I had very little to do with anyone who lived on the street, as they chose not to talk to me or my children. Comments were made to me about being a single parent and not controlling my son. They tried to make life difficult for me by putting notes through my door about my garden being untidy. I did not have the time to spend cutting the grass, or money to buy plants, but I did keep it as tidy as possible. Another thing that made my life difficult was when I couldn't find my rubbish bin because they had moved it. They would not ask about Jonathan or offer any help.

Phoning the police upset me so much, I just felt the whole world was against me and my son. The officer was very understanding and reassured me he would inform the neighbours of my situation and would not expect any more calls of complaints from them. I appreciated his help, but after that morning, it made want to go out less. I felt everyone was talking about me. I was really unhappy that people living around me could go to those lengths because they could not accept my son. I knew I had to try to carry on as best I could. If I stayed in the house hiding, it would not help me or Jonathan; it would be giving in to people who didn't understand.

I had an idea about taking a short bus journey several times a week into town and back. I had to start taking Jonathan into the community more. To try and understand how he saw 'his world.' I got the times of the buses and decided to take an early one at first. Usually there was no one at the bus stop and we would get to the stop with one or two minutes to wait, which was all the time Jonathan would be willing to wait before wanting to go back home. At first, he didn't like it. I would keep talking to him about the shops we would go to. This did not always calm him, especially if other people on the bus were distressing him. I wanted him to try to stay on the bus until we got to town and then come straight back on the next bus if we were not able to go anywhere else, which was very often the case for many weeks. I tried to anticipate problems in order to avoid them if possible. If there was a dog on the bus, we would have to get off straight away and wait for the next bus, or start to walk back home. Having experienced numerous problems trying to complete a short journey. I began to realise what was causing him to become upset. It meant changing the times on certain days or getting off one or two stops before home and walking the rest of the way. I was willing to try everything to help him get used to the bus journey to town and back.

As Jonathan began to cope with going on a bus a few times a week, I tried to build on it by going later in the afternoon, when it was quieter, and also calling into a shop or post office to complete another task and extending his time out of the house.

People who lived near us would see us waiting for the bus or walking home when we got off the bus. They wouldn't speak, only between themselves if there were others there. This was very hurtful. I knew I had to ignore them and keep telling myself that I was helping Jonathan, and that's all that mattered.

When Jonathan had accepted the bus journeys to town and back home, I thought of taking him to our local train station. Again, it would be a different environment and sounds, and he liked his trains. Our first visit to the station was a complete disaster! We had just got through the door and although there were not too many people around, an express train went by very fast and loud. Jonathan was scared, and screamed, and started to run away. I knew I had made the wrong decision. He was not ready for such loud sounds. I took him out straight away and got the next bus home. I needed to keep working on his sensitive hearing. We did not go back to the station for many months. I just stuck with the bus journeys, but with the intention of extending them.

I tried choosing places to visit that may interest both Jonathan and Kelly, hoping she would want to come along too. It would help Jonathan by having his sister with him, and build on their relationship and social skills. I could be with both of my children. Kelly started to make suggestions of visiting a castle or museum, which were good ideas that I could expand on. These trips had to be planned to the last detail. I'd consider the timing of buses, and possible reasons for breaking a journey if Jonathan became distressed. I had to take changes of clothes for him. If he was eating his bread and got bits on his clothes, he would have to change them, or if he spilt his drink of water on his clothes, it would upset him. People around were unkind, and comments made like, 'why don't you change him when you get off?' My reply would be, 'he doesn't understand, and it needs to be done now!' Kelly would feel embarrassed because she could not understand why bits on his clothes or little drops of water caused him to become so upset. I would change him as quickly and calmly as I could but feeling angry inside at the attitude and lack of understanding from people.

I tried not to let incidents like that put me off making sure the children enjoyed their time out. Jonathan was not aware of the prejudice around him because I made sure everything went smoothly. Kelly was noticing how others around us would talk between themselves, or loudly at times, which she said made her want to get off the bus.

When we were going out, Jonathan would take his bread but Kelly liked to stop at McDonald's for some fries. So, as a treat, that is what she had. Each time we went to buy her fries, I would ask Jonathan if he wanted some. As usual he refused. One day Kelly asked for some chicken nuggets, and to my surprise, Jonathan wanted to taste one. Kelly gave him one, and after pulling a face at the different texture, I expected him to throw it away. But no, he ate it! I just couldn't believe what had happened. I was so happy for him. Even though it was just one he had, it was something different. Another small step in his progress that kept me going for another day.

We continued to try going to McDonald's once a week. I would have liked to go more often, but I knew I could not afford it. I would have to cut back on other food items to pay for bus fares and McDonald's food, but I felt the benefits of the whole outing were worth it.

Kelly liked going to museums and castles, and we included her visits as part of her work at home, which I was very pleased about. I managed to get special rates to go into castles when I explained my situation. Very often the staff at the castle or museum would have someone to help Kelly go around with her and explain things to her while I tried to get Jonathan interested in other things. It made me feel I was helping Kelly in a small way to have some quality time for learning. I could not give her that time, but at least I was able to arrange it for her in advance. It took a little of the guilt I felt away from me for a short time.

The day came when I had to make the final payment on the loan I had for the visit to the clinic. Trying to juggle what bills to pay or leave until another time, cutting down on my food, so I could buy the children their food, and extra food for Jonathan to taste. While I felt the visit to the clinic and the programme did help me to understand Jonathan's problems, I knew deep down it was going to take many years to deal with all his issues. I would not be able to go back to the clinic because I could not afford to, but I had 'something' to work on, which I was grateful for.

Over the years, I had been neglecting my own health; not having any time to myself, lack of sleep and food, and the pressure of everyday life. I started getting pains in my chest. I tried to ignore it and took painkiller tablets to get through the days. I began losing the motivation to take Jonathan to the leisure centre as often as I wanted to because I did not have the energy.

Kelly chose to spend more time with her father if we weren't going out. This made me feel I was letting Jonathan down because we could not keep to his routine, which was so important to him. If I felt ill and not able to follow through his usual activities, he got very stressed and his behaviour would become more challenging. At times, if I wasn't able to calm him down, I took him on a short bus journey and straight back.

My health was not improving after a number of weeks, and I was having to take more tablets to take the pain away. I began worrying more about what would happen to Jonathan if I couldn't look after him. At night, if he wouldn't settle in his own room I took him into my room, just so I could get a little sleep. He did seem to like that, which helped me, as I did not have the energy to cope with him getting stressed.

If Kelly was not with her father, she used to comment about Jonathan sleeping in my room, saying, 'He's too old and should be in his own room!'

I was too tired to have to keep explaining how Jonathan was different to her.

A few months had gone by and I was still not getting any better. I knew I had to go and see the doctor. I made an appointment and Jonathan came along with me. Kelly was with her father. In the waiting room Jonathan was starting to get agitated because of the people around him, and there were a few children too. I was experiencing pain in my chest and feeling sick. I went to ask the receptionist how long would I have to wait as I was feeling ill. She said I was next in, which I was grateful for.

The doctor spent a few minutes with me and said without examining me that it was pleurisy and would go in a few weeks. I asked for some stronger painkillers or antibiotics to help me, as I had Jonathan and my daughter to care for.

He could see how Jonathan was behaving and commented, 'You are under a lot of stress, but the pleurisy should clear without antibiotics or strong painkillers.'

He made me feel I was wasting his time and didn't believe what I was telling him. Jonathan and I left the room and went straight home.

I was exhausted, frightened of anything happening to me. Jonathan could not make a phone call to his father or anyone if I needed help. The doctor didn't seem to care about me or the situation I was in. I had no one to turn to for help.

My fears were consuming my every thought. I just wanted to sleep, and that night Jonathan slept alongside me, and he slept what seemed like all night, waking at 4 a.m.

I was having to reduce the number of journeys out of the house. The cough I started developing was making the pains in my chest worse. My long hair was falling out too, and my weight was dropping. I knew I needed help but had nowhere to turn to. After months of trying to cope with my health getting worse, I was becoming desperate. I was extremely tired, very depressed and fearful for my life. My thoughts were consumed with the worry: 'what will happen to Jonathan?' I knew my daughter would be looked after by her father, but I did not feel he could cope or understand Jonathan's needs.

I decided to make another appointment with the doctor to try to get some medication. Again, he said he could not give me anything. I explained that my cough was getting worse and I was coughing up blood. The chest pains I had was causing me concern. He decided to refer me to a heart specialist and informed me that the waiting time to see one would be at least four months.

I left the surgery feeling more down and in despair!

Doing any routine chores was becoming difficult. All I could focus on was getting Jonathan's meals. Kelly was at her father's more, which reassured me she was doing her work. It was Jonathan I felt guilty about; not being able to keep up with his activities he needed to do.

Life was looking bleak. With no hope of improving and with my health deteriorating, I felt as though I had reached the end of the road. I was starting to think about ending my life and my son's. If I was diagnosed with a heart problem, I knew I would not be able to care for Jonathan as he needed. With the love I had for my son, I knew he would have to be with me.

I began planning in my head and going over everything when one day there was a knock at the door. I wasn't expecting anyone, as no one came to visit. It was two young women, who said they were missionaries in the area, and asked if they could help in any way.

I hadn't heard from my church since Jonathan's christening at three months old. They said they were not from my church. I decided to let them in, because I needed to talk to someone. I explained the situation, and they offered to visit regularly and bring food, and to carry out any chores that needed doing, without any obligations or pressure. They just wanted to help. I was so moved by their kindness I accepted their offer of help. Jonathan accepted them being in the house too. They called several times a week and prepared Jonathan's food, did some cleaning, and put washing in the machine. I was so grateful I had someone who wanted to help, but I knew I could not rely on or expect it for too long as they would be moving on, which they did after a number of weeks.

My health was still not improving. It was clear the pains in my chest were due to a heart problem. My long hair was falling out in handfuls. I was frightened to brush it. I was coughing up blood and my weight was down to six stone. I knew I was desperately ill and didn't know what to do. The appointment with the specialist had not come through yet.

Thoughts of ending it all were at the front of my mind. I had to do it while I had the strength, which I felt would not be for too long.

Kelly was at home the morning I feared the worst was happening to me. It was a strange and frightening feeling, which I can only describe as an out-of-body experience. I remember looking at the clock and it was 7 a.m. Jonathan was lying beside me, awake but not moving, just looking at me. I tried to get up out of bed but I couldn't move. Then something really strange happened. I was looking down on myself from high above, with Jonathan lying beside me. I remember saying out loud, 'I've got to get him his drink of milk!' It seemed as though I had left my physical body, and I was scared because I knew I had to look after Jonathan. When I looked at the clock again, it was still 7 a.m. I called out to Kelly, who came into the room looking confused. I asked her to phone her father and tell him that he needed to come over and then phone the emergency number for an ambulance because I needed a doctor. She came back to say her father was not there, but the ambulance was coming. My mind went into practical mode. I asked her to get Jonathan his drink of milk and open the front door. Jonathan stayed very close to me when the paramedics came into the room.

I explained how I had been and that I needed some painkillers. They wanted me to go to hospital, but I couldn't. I just needed to rest. As it was a child phoning for an ambulance, a policeman called out too and asked for the address of the children's father. They went round to inform him that he needed to take care of the children. I said I just needed a day or two to rest and something to take the pain away. I had to let Kelly and Jonathan stay with their father for a few days, even though he didn't have much room at his flat. I was worried about Jonathan and how stressful he would find it. But I had no choice. I never mentioned this experience to anyone through fear of ridicule.

After a rest for two days, the pain had eased a little and Kelly and Jonathan came back home. Their father was rather agitated and had not been coping with Jonathan's behaviour. He didn't offer to have them both together again, but said he would pick up Kelly later that week. I could see Jonathan was upset, because he was out of his normal routine and it would take time for him to settle.

I was able to function a little more because I was in less pain. But I realised my situation was not good, and the children's father had not coped with Jonathan. This all compounded the fears I had for the future.

The appointment to see the heart specialist arrived. I asked the children's father if he could look after both of them while I went to the hospital. I could not say how long it would take. He agreed, which helped to take the stress off me. I got to the appointment and had to wait half an hour to see the doctor. When I went into the room, I noticed how smartly dressed he was, with a bright red fancy bow tie. He asked me a few questions and said it was not a heart problem, just pleurisy, and I was young enough to get over it. He came across as uncaring and arrogant. I just got up and left the room; relieved it wasn't a heart problem, but scared because I did not know what it was.

Walking out of the hospital, I crossed the road and saw a bus coming that went into Birmingham. Something told me to get on the bus and go to the Chinese Herbal Medicine Clinic. I knew where it was, having passed it every day when I worked in Birmingham. I felt a strange need to go there. Not checking if I had enough money for the fare, I put my hand out to stop the bus. After asking the driver how much the fare was to Birmingham, he said it was a special rate after 10 a.m. I had enough money! I kept thinking to myself all the way there, 'if they can't help me, I'm finished.'

When I got to the clinic and walked in, I explained I did not have an appointment, having just come from the hospital. The two doctors there were so kind and helpful. They told me not to worry and to sit down, then offered me a glass of water and said they would talk with me when they had finished with a patient.

I went into the consulting room, where I gave the doctors details of my condition and how long it had been going on. They were shocked by the attitude of the specialist and my GP.

After taking various tests, including on my hair, they explained that my whole immune system had broken down and would take a very long time to recover. The herbal medicine they were going to give me would need to be boiled in water and drunk several times a day. I asked how much it would cost. To my amazement and shock, they said, they would not accept any money. They wanted to help me!

I was overcome with emotion and couldn't thank them enough. I took the bags of herbs and agreed to let them know how I was after a week. I looked at the time, surprised to find I had been there two hours, and made my way back home, relieved someone had taken me seriously and given me an explanation that I understood,

I started to think over. Why couldn't my doctor or specialist help me but a doctor in alternative medicine felt they could? My trust in our healthcare system had gone.

I was still in pain and feeling nauseous coughing up blood, but determined to try the herbal medicine.

Jonathan came back that evening tired, upset, and stressed at not being in his routine. Kelly was staying with her father. I was too tired to question their father why she hadn't come home. He left straight away after dropping Jonathan off. To try and settle Jonathan I put on his *Thomas the Tank Engine* videos while I boiled my first cup of herbal medicine. I could only take it a teaspoonful at a time.

I was not expecting any great improvements to happen quickly, but at least I had something that was going to build up my immune system and help me to eat again. I knew my weight was getting dangerously low. After the first week of taking the herbal medicine, my cough was easing up. I was still having to take painkillers, but I was able keep the medicine down. I phoned the clinic to let them know and they were pleased with the results. As they had given me a four-week supply of herbs, they asked me to complete the course and visit them again when I could after that.

My energy levels were very low and I could not do very much of Jonathan's programme. I had the idea of trying to get him to sit at the table and start learning to write the alphabet. I felt I had to keep doing something to help him. I put the pen in his hand to write the letter A, and complete the alphabet. Then I held his hand to guide the pen to write his name. He would only cooperate for about ten to fifteen minutes at a time, but it was a start. I did this for two or three times a day, every day. I carried on until he could follow the letters himself. To begin with, he was writing one letter on an A4 piece of paper. It filled the whole page. When he managed to do all of the alphabet on a page for each letter, I would go over them three, four, five times a day, trying to get him to say or make the sound of each letter. I didn't know if he would be able to understand but I had to keep trying, however long it took him to learn. If he could grasp his letters, I could build on that by forming simple words for him to read, like train, cup, cat, ball. It felt like the right place to start, and it would help me to understand how he saw letters.

It was giving me a goal to work towards and taking my mind off my health issues. Deep down I knew my son had the ability to understand, if only I could find a way of helping him. That fear of him being institutionalised by the age of ten or eleven years old was always tormenting me and driving me to keep going.

Over the weeks of not being able to go out much because of my health, while completing the course of herbal medicine I spent a lot of time with Jonathan, helping him write the alphabet, his name and a few simple words. I was amazed and so happy when he started saying the letters and words. I knew if he could start to make the sounds, he would be able to talk. These steps of progress meant the world to me. Although he was approaching eight years old and not developing as a child without autism would be expected to, it made me very happy that the signs of his capability were there. I began to think to myself, 'what does it matter if he can't talk, or dress, or wash himself for his age? I could teach him to, however long it takes!'

I finished my course of herbal medicine and had to arrange to go back to the clinic. I had to ask the children's father to look after them both as I had an appointment. The journey was exhausting and the walk from the bus stop was very difficult, but I was determined to do it. The doctors at the clinic were worried that I hadn't made as much progress as expected. I explained I was reducing the number of painkillers I was taking, but I couldn't eat anything yet. They were shocked I had made the journey on my own by bus. They said I must go home by taxi. Having explained my situation and lack of money they informed me they would arrange a taxi to take me back and give me more herbs for two months. This kind gesture overwhelmed me, and I got very upset. I asked if I was going to get better. They advised me to complete the next course of medicine and phone in once a week to let them know how I was doing. I accepted their offer of a taxi home. It was very much appreciated as I was feeling quite ill and knew I might not be able to cope with the long bus journey home.

Having got home much sooner than I expected, I did not phone the children's father straight away to say bring them back. I just wanted a little time on my own.

I was starting to realise how desperate the situation was becoming, and fearing my health would not improve. Jonathan had so many issues to deal with, and little hope of any future, I felt absolute despair. There did not seem to be any hope of life getting better. What was the point of it all?

After a short rest I phoned to say I was back home, and the children could be brought home. I was pleased that Kelly came home too. Although we were not close anymore, I felt guilty about the difficult situation she was having to deal with. She spent a lot of time in her room, which I accepted as her way of getting some time and space to herself. Jonathan got back into his routine, which calmed him down.

As I could only manage a short journey to shop once a week because of my health condition, I had to go by taxi as I would not be able to cope with going on a bus. The cost put yet more strain on my finances, but I was cutting back on items to pay for it. I kept thinking, if I could get through the next two months taking the herbal medicine, I may be able to go by bus again.

Each day I kept trying to focus on Jonathan doing his sensory programme and writing the alphabet and a few simple words. Still introducing a new taste of food with his pasta, I managed to buy some frozen chicken nuggets from the supermarket, which he was willing to eat one or two of.

The sound tape was part of his daily routine, and it did seem to be calming him down. Routine had to be followed rigidly. Whatever I introduced into his day or night, after a while, had to be kept going. Mealtimes were set too. Along with the alphabet, I had the idea of helping him to tell the time. He understood certain times of the day, that breakfast was at 5 a.m., lunchtime at noon, pasta at 4 p.m. I was sure he could be taught about the clock. I started drawing clocks with his mealtimes on and showing him the picture. I also took the clock off the wall each time to reenforce what time it is. He picked that up very quickly and was starting to say 5 o'clock; not clearly, but enough for me to know he was understanding.

When he watched his *Thomas the Tank Engine* videos, it gave me another idea of using trains as a way of helping him to learn the time. Over many weeks I would draw clocks with different times on; just working on each hour at first and going over them several times a day. Along with his alphabet and words, he was spending more time learning things that he could relate to in his world. This was also helping me to find other ways of teaching him, by involving things that he was interested in, and I could expand on as we went on.

I tried not to build up my hopes too much, because I was not sure how my health would be. I took my herbal medicine each day, but there was not as much improvement as I thought there would be.

Maybe I expected too much. After all, the specialist couldn't help, so how was the herbal medicine going to? It was all I had, and I hoped it would.

As time passed, my cough was slowing down and I was able to eat small amounts of food. The pain was still quite bad, but I was taking fewer tablets for the pain. I didn't have much energy, but I was doing what I could each day.

I made sure Jonathan kept trying to learn a little with his reading and writing, and speech skills. Kelly was spending more time with her father doing her work. I felt guilty not being able to do more. As a mother, I was pleased by how intelligent she was, and would grow up to lead her own life. My worries and fears were for Jonathan's future. More now if my health didn't improve. The dark thoughts started to come into my mind again,

I was losing contact with my daughter, who did not want to be with me. She was not able to relate to her brother. I knew how far ahead she was at ten years old compared to Jonathan, who at eight years old, couldn't talk, wash or dress himself. He was engrossed with playing on his own with his trains. Any tiny glimpse of progress Jonathan seemed to be making, to me, was all the hope I had, and it made me want to keep trying, even though it seemed hopeless.

I finished the two months' supply of herbal medicine, and I was feeling a little better. I phoned the clinic to book another appointment, as I felt I could make the bus journey there and back. The children stayed with their father. The doctors were pleased with my improvement, but still felt it was going to take time for me to regain my health and weight. They gave me more packets of herbs for another month. I accepted on the condition that they would have the money from me.

With the loan paid off, I was starting to clear some of the bills slowly. I wanted to pay for my medicine. I was very grateful for their kindness, and I wanted to contribute to my herbs. I managed to get home without feeling too tired, and I felt that was progress. I realised I had pushed myself too much over the years, and my body just broke down. I had to look after myself if I was going to be there for Jonathan.

I was starting to appreciate how herbal medicine was helping me. That day coming out of the hospital after seeing the specialist, and the strange feeling I had to get the bus to Birmingham, to go to an herbalist clinic that I knew was there but had never been in, turned out to be the treatment that saved my life.

As I was reaching a stage where I could eat small amounts of different foods and the pain was easing, I knew I had to make sure I did not over do anything, as it was going to take time to fully recover, once the herbal medicine had helped to build up my immune system.

During those months, Jonathan continued learning the alphabet and writing it out. I carried on drawing clocks and encouraged him to put the numbers on, and different times. This activity expanded to him counting up to twelve at first so he could relate the numbers to the clock time. We did a few each day and repeated saying the time several times during the day. I was beginning to understand where his difficulties were and took it all very slowly, not moving on with anything new until I felt he had understood each step. It took many months of working on the time and each day drawing clocks, and encouraging him to put the numbers on, then different times.

His speech was starting to improve a little and his behaviour was becoming more manageable. Even though Jonathan had developmental delay in many areas of his life, he was showing me he *could* learn. That made me determined to try to help him, with a great deal of love, time and patience, encouraging him in each new task he was learning. I was trying to understand how he saw things and finding different ways to help him.

The challenge before me was enormous. I had to accept as a mother that my son needed help to learn and do just about everything if he was going to have any quality of life. Apart from learning to read and write, he wasn't able to have a bath or shower, brush his teeth, couldn't dress himself or put shoes on, and his lack of appetite or willingness to try other foods was a constant struggle. His sensory and coordination problems affected his daily life. His need to stick rigidly to his routine meant everything had to be planned around what was important to *him*. His lack of verbal communication made it extremely difficult at times to know what was upsetting him at that moment.

Another area of his autism that I was aware of and which worried me greatly, was his lack of imagination. He preferred to be on his own with his trains. I found it hard to get him to play with other toys, like cars or boats. When I tried to interact and encourage playing, pretending to be a lion and making the sound of a lion, or any other animal, Jonathan had to go back to his trains, because he could not understand 'pretend play.' He related to his trains because he saw them on his *Thomas the Tank Engine* videos that he watched over and over, and would want to take his trains everywhere with him. When we went shopping, he would have to take his trains with him. People used to look at him, and at times make comments I could hear, such as, 'he's a bit old for that.' Although Jonathan was nine years old, he was not mentally aware and did not understand. I did not want to upset him by not letting him take them, but I understood I needed to help him 'grow up' and wean him off them.

Jonathan was not developing as you would expect a child without problems to. Therefore, he wouldn't understand what behaviour issues were not considered 'normal' for a certain age in development.

There were so many problems I knew I had to work on with him. The responsibility was overwhelming, and many times I did not feel I was able to cope with such a difficult challenge.

Being out of the system meant we were isolated. Not having any contact with other parents or children with similar issues, I had to try and make sense of it all myself and find a way of coping. I knew this was going to be a very long, ongoing challenge. As his mother, the love and protection of my son gave me the strength and determination to try to help him.

In another year, Jonathan would be ten years old. I never forgot that statement made by the therapists at the clinic we visited, saying if I didn't do something now, Jonathan would be institutionalised by the age of ten or eleven. The fear of that happening stayed with me, and I knew if I could get him to that age with the little steps of progress he was making, maybe there was a chance of him improving more.

Over the following year I continued to work on the things that were helping him to calm down, which then enabled me to work on other issues. I continued to work with him doing the alphabet, reading and writing, introducing different smells and sounds and learning to tell the time. I felt that dealing with some of his issues over time and getting small steps of progress, was proving more achievable than trying to work on all areas.

Chapter Three
Ten to Fifteen Years Old

Continuing to work on Jonathan's sensory issues, along with his reading, writing and learning to tell the time, I knew I had to try to encourage him to sleep in his own bedroom by himself. Although it was going to be difficult; it was a part of his development that I needed to help him with before he got any older. As a mother, I knew if Jonathan was going to live any kind of 'normal' life, he had to be encouraged in his maturing.

I decided to stay with him for an hour when he went to bed. I would read books with him and talk about him going to sleep when I left the room. I reassured him everything was alright, and he could have his bedside lamp light on. I also reminded him to go to the toilet. At first, when I left his room, he would get up straight away and come into my room. I then explained it was time to go back to bed and was not breakfast time yet. After taking him back to his room, I only stayed for a few minutes before leaving. This encouragement took many weeks before he got to the stage when he was able to stay in his room for an hour or so; if he got up to go to the toilet, he would want to go downstairs to watch his videos. He thought when he got up to go to the toilet it was time to 'get up', whatever the time was! I knew this process would take time for him to adjust to, as it was difficult for him to understand day and night. I had to keep trying, even though it meant him starting his day at three or four in the morning. I accepted he would not stay in his room any longer and would start getting stressed and loud.

My daughter was spending more time with her father, which meant she wasn't being disturbed early in the mornings. I could concentrate on encouraging Jonathan with his development.

I was becoming concerned about Kelly not being with other children. When she did come home for a few days at a time, she didn't seem to want to talk to me or Jonathan. If I asked her about her work, she would not want to say much. I felt she needed to go back into school. Her social skills were being affected. I had to accept my time was taken up with looking after Jonathan, who was becoming calmer and manageable in his behaviour. I tried to explain to Kelly that he was staying in his own bedroom, learning new skills, and making progress. I asked her to stay with us longer so she could see how Jonathan was changing and to come out on a day trip with us. Kelly did not seem interested in any of my suggestions. I approached the subject of her going back into school and explained that because Jonathan was autistic and needed a great deal of support, our family life was difficult. I suggested that she talk with her friends and ask them about the school they go to, then she could join them and feel part of a 'normal' life. I was hoping she would think about it. I decided the next time I took her to the groups; I would mention schools to the parents of her friends, and ask them to let Kelly know how they get on there. I felt the time was right for her to be back in school.

My physical health was improving. I was getting to the stage of not having to take the Chinese herbal medicine, and I could eat a small amount of food. I was able to get a few hours' sleep, as Jonathan progressed with his bedtime routine. I accepted a 3 or 4 a.m. start to the day was the best solution to avoid causing Jonathan or myself any more added stress. He did not need very much sleep, which I realised must be part of his autism. I was making sure he was mentally active with the different skills we were doing, but I felt he needed to do more physical activities, which I couldn't do yet, as my health was not at a stage for overdoing things.

Although Jonathan's behaviour was improving, he was still not able to cope with new challenges. Everything had to be taken at his pace of coping.

After picking up Kelly from her group one day, she came out with a surprise statement. She said, 'I want to go back into school, the one that my friends go to.'

I was so pleased to hear her say that, even though I knew it would be difficult at first for her, having been out of school for a number of years. I felt confident she would settle back in and not be behind with her work.

I contacted the school she chose and took her along to see the head teacher. I explained our family situation, and how Kelly was keeping up with her work at home. The head teacher was understanding and agreed to accept Kelly into the school. After looking round the school and completing the necessary paperwork, knowing Kelly felt happy about going was a huge relief for me. Hopefully she would begin to feel some normality in her life. Going on the school bus, as the school was out of our area, would give her a little independence too.

Kelly settled into school and was doing well. The teachers were pleased with how much work she had done, and was far ahead intellectually for her age, approaching twelve years old.

I was able to continue encouraging Jonathan without worrying too much about Kelly, as her teachers recognised her ability and were helping her as much as possible.

I realised I needed to start taking Jonathan out again. He had got used to being in the house. Although he had been working on his different activities with me, we had been confined to the home for some time as a result of my health, which was improving slowly. I had an idea to try to help him with telling the time. We would visit our local railway station. It had been a long time since our last unsuccessful attempt. I felt I needed to try again to see if Jonathan could cope, having worked on his auditory sense for some time now.

I talked to Jonathan about going on the bus to the train station and look at the trains. Reassuring him we would only stay for a short while and go back home. I suggested that he take one of his toy trains to encourage him to go. I needed to try this experience again.

When we got off the bus and walked to the station, Jonathan was calm. I talked about the trains, ticket office, guards and the clock. We went through the doors and passed the ticket office, before I started showing him the different things at a station, like on his *Thomas the Tank Engine* videos. Then we went outside onto the platform. I pointed out the clock, and when an announcement came over the speaker to say what time the next train would be arriving. I kept his attention on the clock as it changed the minutes. Keeping him calm was difficult, but I wanted him to stay and see the train. He was scared of the noise, so I put my hands over his ears. As the train pulled up slowly, I took my hands down to see if he could cope. To my surprise he did cope for a minute or two, then we had to leave. I was so pleased the experience was not as frightening as the first visit. Even though it was a short visit, I knew he had overcome another hurdle and it was something I could build on, as I was always striving to do.

On the way back home, I talked about the experience and how we could go again. To my surprise, he was not stressed about the idea. There was something else I noticed but did not bring his attention to: he had not taken his train out of his pocket since leaving home or arriving back. I felt deep down that this experience had helped him more than I expected, but I didn't want to get my hopes up too much!

We started to make regular visits to the train station, staying a little longer each time. Jonathan was getting used to the different sounds, and if the noise was uncomfortable for him, I would encourage him to put his hands up to his ears and take them down when he felt ready to. This also helped me to observe how he was coping in the environment. I intended to build on this experience and make a short train journey when Jonathan was able to cope with the idea.

As we did with the bus journeys, taking it gradually and at Jonathan's pace, I found the train times that would be twenty minutes to the next nearest town. This would also help him to become familiar with the place names he could hear over the speaker. I kept talking about the time and pointing to the station clock, showing how the minutes changed. I knew he was interested, and it was an idea I had when drawing clocks with him: we could now put on the minutes too and build on it. I was always trying to think of ways that would help him.

When the day came that we were going to make a short train journey, I had checked every detail to ensure it would be successful. As the train pulled into the station and the doors opened, Jonathan was a little anxious about getting on. I knew we only had a few minutes to decide what we were going to do. I was expecting Jonathan to want to go home, when a guard came up to us and said in a pleasant manner, 'The train will be leaving in one minute, if you want to get on.'

I looked at Jonathan's face, and he said, 'One minute.' Then he stepped onto the train. I was so surprised and happy that *he* had made the decision about getting on. He sat and looked out of the window. I was talking about the different things we saw. There were not too many people on the train, which helped him cope with the journey. When we got to our destination, he remembered the station name he heard over the speaker. We got off and as I had planned, waited for the next train back, which was on time and only a few minutes' wait. The experience went very well for Jonathan, and I felt relieved and happy that he coped far better than I could have expected. Again, although he had his train in his pocket, he didn't take it out. I felt that with him experiencing real trains, this would in time help Jonathan not rely on his toy trains.

I started drawing the minutes on his clocks and going over it several times each day, and it amazed me how quickly he was picking it up. I thought I was going to confuse him when we had to go past twelve o'clock. As train timetables work on the twenty-four-hour clock. I had to show him that after twelve o'clock noon, it was thirteen hundred hours, fourteen, fifteen and so on up until midnight. He had difficulty understanding that after midnight it started again at 1 a.m.

I had to find a way of helping him understand. It took several weeks encouraging him to draw clocks and going over the times and minutes on the clocks, which he liked doing. When we got to saying twelve night time, I tried explaining that another starts, and we say 1 a.m., and go round the clock again until midnight. To show him, we would go to the railway station at different times, so he could see the clock before midday and afternoon. We would also do a short train journey at different times to help him understand. It was something I could visualise that we could build on, and he could learn a great deal from over time. I felt I had got an interest Jonathan enjoyed, and it would help him with his transition from his toy trains, to experiencing real-life trains and people. This was a turning point in his development, because I now knew he had the ability to learn. That comment about how he would no doubt be institutionalised had been proven wrong.

I was gaining more confidence with taking him out, and his behaviour was becoming more manageable for me. I could anticipate possible problems that may cause him anxiety and either try to avoid them, help Jonathan cope with situations that were difficult, or take him out of the environment.

I experienced hurtful comments from people at railways, shops and society in general. If he was getting stressed about something, my only concern was to try to calm him down and find out the problem, which was not always easy. I was aware people were looking at us, or would move away from us, but that did not embarrass me; it made me realise society had no understanding of what being autistic meant. The distress Jonathan would show when he was frightened about something he did not understand and could not verbally communicate was not bad behaviour, as it would be judged as.

I continued with the train journeys and extending the time before we got the next train back home. We would sometimes call at McDonald's for his chicken nuggets. I wanted to keep trying to get him to eat one or two, and hopefully to build on this by one day sitting down to eat them inside the café instead of our usual routine of being served quickly and taking the food outside to eat, before getting on the train home. I was always thinking of different ideas to help him to cope in the 'real' world.

His lack of sleep and early start to each day meant he would usually be watching his videos for hours. Since visiting the railway station and going on the trains, he chose not to watch his *Thomas the Tank Engine* videos. I encouraged him to watch other videos that helped with his reading, counting and colours. I used to hire them from the library at a very reasonable cost and could swap them each week. To my amazement, Jonathan took an interest in the new videos. Another huge step in his developmental progress that gave me hope that I was going in the right direction with him.

I was pleased to find out that a McDonald's food outlet would be opening not too far from where we lived, and the times of opening would be from 6 a.m. My thoughts turned to going for a walk with Jonathan. It would be exercise for us both, and quiet at that time of day. Hopefully the physical activity would help improve his sleep too. I talked about it with Jonathan when McDonald's opened, suggesting he went for a drink of milk or water. As it was summer and light in the mornings, it would be a pleasant walk. I didn't expect him to go inside for a drink but was hoping he would for a rest. Our first visit meant leaving the house after he had breakfast and being at McDonald's at 6 a.m. We went in to a buy drink but he didn't want to sit down. He took his bottle of water to drink on the way home. Although I was tired, and he wanted to start walking straight back, I was pleased with the way he coped with this new experience, and I felt confident it could be built on with time, with him sitting down to have a drink, and maybe some toast. My intention was to try doing this once a week, as it would take time to eventually build his confidence to sit inside to eat. I knew it had to be done at Jonathan's pace.

Throughout the summer months, we walked once a week to McDonald's early in the morning, even though it was just to go in and purchase his drink of milk or bottle of water and make our way back home. I had no idea how long it would take, if ever, for Jonathan to sit down to eat or drink inside, but I felt it had benefits to his physical health by walking, and I was prepared to carry on doing this as long as he wanted to.

As time passed from summer to autumn, and winter to spring, we were able to experience the changes in the weather and talk about it. Also, the need to wear warm clothing as the weather got colder. It was difficult to motivate myself to do the walk in the cold, dark mornings, but it helped Jonathan to learn about the seasons. It was the best way for him to understand by getting wet in the rain, walking in the snow, strong winds, seeing the leaves fall off the trees. He could see and experience the changes for himself.

I was learning to understand how *he* understood his environment, and how I could develop those experiences further. Bringing up a child without autism or any kind of learning disability, we expect them to get to a certain age and assume they will just learn about their environment. With Jonathan and his complex issues, he had to be shown and taught in a different way, as his way of thinking and understanding requires tremendous patience, visual and sensory learning, which I was starting to realise more.

My thoughts and concerns turned to Kelly and her behaviour, which was starting to make me feel unsettled. She was doing very well at school, but she had given up her drama and dance groups. Her reasons were her lack of time after school, due to homework. I accepted her reasons, but tried to explain to her that it was important to have other interests outside of school. As Kelly had given up going to her groups it meant she would be able to spend more time with her father during the week. I felt it was another way of moving further away from me! But in a way, I felt I somehow deserved it. Her father was agreeable with Kelly's decisions, and considered her schoolwork more important than drama or dance groups. My opinion did not seem to matter. I had to accept what they chose to do.

I knew Kelly was progressing intellectually, but her attitude towards her brother and myself, worried me. She would not accept that I loved them both and the talents they each had. As a result of the care one needed, the ability of the other, and lack of support as a family, our lives could never be what society considered 'normal'.

I had to accept my daughter did not want to be part of mine or Jonathan's life. Maybe, it was her blaming me for what she considered as me 'spoiling' him, and hoping one day Jonathan would be 'normal'. I could not stand in the way of her education. Her father was giving her the support and time she needed. Contact with school became scarce over time, as all reports were sent to her father on his request. As a mother, I felt a complete failure. I wanted so much to be part of my daughter's life as well as my son's. Deep down I felt emotionally torn apart. I did not want Kelly growing up thinking people who have autism or any kind of disability were considered not worthwhile. Sadly, I was not given the opportunity to influence her growing up.

Going for our walk early mornings to McDonald's, and experiencing the change of seasons, Jonathan could see the signs of spring, as we walked past gardens and could see the daffodils growing. He was very interested in seeing the flowers starting to grow and could relate them to the weather changing. The snow had gone, the frosty mornings would soon be gone, and summer would begin. I talked about different clothes to wear when it was hot, and how we would not need to put on a coat or gloves. I tried to turn every experience into an opportunity to learn. Even though we had started our early-morning walk to McDonald's the previous summer, it was now almost spring. Jonathan had not yet reached the stage of wanting to sit inside to have his drink or something to eat. I was still hopeful by the time summer was here, he would feel comfortable about eating inside. It had to be when *he* was ready.

We continued to do the train journeys and working on telling the time, which Jonathan was making progress with. His reading and writing skills were improving, and his sensory issues by introducing different smells and sounds. I had stopped using the auditory tape gradually over time, as we were going to the railway station more.

He started coping with the different sounds and would choose to put his hands over his ears if he thought he couldn't cope. This was showing me he knew what sounds were too loud for him, like express trains. When he heard over the speaker that one would be passing through, he could prepare himself. It also meant he was listening to the announcements, as I tried to remind him to do, to learn about different destinations and times. This was wonderful progress, and something we could further expand on.

His sensitivity to smells still needed to be worked on. When we were out and passed a coffee shop, the smell of coffee made him nauseous. Similarly, if we were on a train and someone was drinking coffee near to where we were sitting, Jonathan would start to feel nauseous, so I used to carry a bottle of aromatherapy oil that he liked and would ask him to smell it and breathe slowly, hoping it would help the sensation pass. Again, I had to be prepared and try to anticipate possible problems that would cause him to become stressed and anxious.

Jonathan's communication skills were just one or two words to express his needs. He was reading short sentences from books he liked and recognised a variety of words that he looked at each day. I would write words like train, cup, bed, bus, spoon and ball out on individual cards; they were objects or things that had a meaning to *him*. Although he was beginning to read short sentences, he could not speak in sentences. This was a constant worry for me. I didn't understand; if he could speak the words when reading, why couldn't he put more words together when talking or asking for something? I knew I had to keep trying with his reading skills in order to help his speech, as his communication skills were so limited for a child approaching eleven years old.

My motivation and determination to try and understand how Jonathan learnt new things meant having an enormous amount of patience and time, not to rush him or assume he had understood a certain task, just because he had said 'yes' to something. I had to make sure over and over again he understood what I was trying to show him by putting it in a different way to him. For example, if I asked him whether he wanted to go on the train, he would say yes. If I asked him whether he wanted to go on an express train, he would also say yes. I knew he didn't fully understand what the question about an express train meant; he just picked up on the word 'train'. Knowing he would not like to go on an express train, I realised when asking him a question I had to use words that he could relate to, to find out what his needs and wants were.

Jonathan had the ability to learn and was proving that in all he was achieving. He was learning to tell the time, and understanding the twenty-four-hour clock that railway timetables work to. He was reading words he could relate to. These achievements were giving me hope he could learn more. I had to keep trying for my son's sake.

My thoughts were never far from wondering how Kelly was doing. I tried very hard not to dwell on Jonathan's developmental delay compared to Kelly, who was exceptionally intelligent for her age, approaching thirteen years old. She hardly came to visit Jonathan and me, using her schoolwork as the reason. I tried to explain how Jonathan was progressing and he would like to see her more often, but no promises were made by her to arrange to do so.

I knew deep inside I must accept the blame as a mother. My life had changed forever after Jonathan was ill with the virus. I knew it had affected him, but no one would listen to me. My love for my son and drive to help him had caused both the breakdown of my relationship with the children's father and for my daughter to feel left out in place of her brother, who had so many complex issues. I was a single parent with no support and very little money trying to deal with two children with different needs. The family life I had wanted so much had turned into an impossible nightmare.

The only comforting thoughts I had to hold onto were that my daughter had a future and my son was able to learn.

I started thinking of other ways to help Jonathan with his coordination skills, as we weren't going to the leisure centre anymore. I decided to try him with learning to ride a bike. I couldn't afford to buy one but knew of a cycle hire shop near our town. After making enquiries and finding out the costs, which were very reasonable, I talked to Jonathan to see if he would like to try it. I knew just explaining would not be enough to help him understand, so we went along to the shop, where they showed him the different bikes and the cycle track nearby for him to use. He wasn't happy about getting on a bike at the first visit, but when he went again, he was anxious but willing to try.

The assistant was helpful and understanding, and walked by him, holding onto the bike until Jonathan began to feel comfortable and steady. I was confident he could ride by himself, again proving his coordination problems were improving. Every new skill Jonathan was learning was keeping me going and wanting to give him every opportunity to develop.

It was only after a few visits to the cycle hire track that Jonathan was riding confidently by himself. I felt so happy for him because I knew he felt as though he had achieved something, and clearly enjoyed doing it. This was an activity that could be expanded with time.

With the few hours of sleep Jonathan was getting, and staying in his own room, it gave me some time to think over the progress he was making doing the different activities. I had to plan how to include tasks that would give him not just mental stimulation, but physical too.

I was aware that other issues needed to be worked on before he got to an age when I would find it more challenging to deal with, like being able to wash or shower himself, or dress and change his clothes. The fact that he could not take care of his personal hygiene without support worried me greatly; it would bring to mind the fears I had for his future. Who would care for him when I was not there? I started to feel angry with myself for not dealing with the problems sooner. I felt I had failed Jonathan.

Whenever he had a bath or shower, I had to make sure the water was not too hot or cold. He wasn't aware of the danger. But the time had come when I had to find a way of teaching him. I knew the process was going to take time, and that he might never manage doing it all, but I wanted him to gain as much independence as possible within his capabilities.

I started asking him to help me with filling the bath water, talking about how warm or cold it felt to him and getting him to put his hand in to feel it. Sometimes I would cool it down to see if he could feel the different temperature, then warm it up again with hot water and ask him to feel it. To begin with Jonathan wasn't aware of what I was showing him; being used to just getting into the bath after I had prepared it. Now I was breaking the process down into stages, though he couldn't understand why. After many times of going through with him how to fill a bath safely, I began encouraging him to wash his hair; helping him with how much shampoo to use and how to rinse it properly, and always talking to him about taking care of his body. I would let him carry out the process as much as he could, with me finishing it if he got stressed. After showing him how to wash his body and rinse the soap off, he had to learn how to dry himself properly; first getting out of the bath safely. To begin with Jonathan did not want to cooperate and would try to get out of the bathroom. I knew I had to somehow encourage him, and I could not put off this issue any longer.

As a mother who was devoted to helping her son, I did not want him being totally dependent on someone else to wash and dress him for the rest of his life. I would teach him, however long it took! It was more added stress to my daily life, and many times I asked myself how much more I could take.

After many frustrating months of helping Jonathan with his self-care skills, I was doubting if he would ever be able to bathe himself, when one day he said, 'bath time!' He quite happily helped to fill the bath, and remembered he must test the temperature, which I supervised, and he got all the things he needed. This made me very happy, because he was choosing to do it himself!

We went through the routine of washing his hair, then he said, 'Jonathan do it.' He wanted to carry on washing himself. I decided it was safe for me to leave the room for a few minutes and let him have his independence. I was standing behind the door in case he needed help

I could hear him going through the process, saying out loud, 'Neck, arms, body, legs and out.' Then he got out safely and dried himself, before calling out, 'All done, finished.' I went into the bathroom trying not to sound too excited, and praised him on how well he had done by himself.

It was signs of improvements like these that not only kept me going when I just couldn't see any point to, but that were proving, however difficult life was for me, that Jonathan was capable of *more*. I just had to keep trying. His self-care skills would have to be encouraged for the foreseeable future, but he'd got to the stage of understanding that he must wash himself, which was another hurdle he had overcome.

Dressing and undressing would also be an ongoing issue that needed to be worked on. Finding clothes made of soft materials that he could tolerate wearing was tricky. He was also not able to tie shoelaces, and after trying different ways to help him to do them, he still could not manage it. I accepted it would always be a problem for him, so I had to look for footwear that he could put on himself that did not have laces. Buttons and zips were also difficult for Jonathan to do even though I used to get him to try and do several times a day. Nonetheless, I felt with continual practice, his dexterity would improve.

He was making a little progress with his food, having cereal or toasted brown bread occasionally for breakfast, and chicken nuggets, fries, beans, eggs, pasta or sausages for his lunch or dinner. Although anything he ate was not in great amounts, it was an improvement from only eating white bread and pasta. I realised his appetite and tastes were a complicated issue, one which I felt was going to be difficult to make any changes to until Jonathan was willing.

I was not going to rush him or expect him to have a wide choice of foods. I was prepared to stay with what he liked and would eat, rather than risk him not eating, as he did when we visited the clinic, and they didn't have any white bread or pasta. Jonathan refused to eat at all. I will never forget that experience.

He liked his food set out on his plate in a certain way; if there were different foods on his plate, they could not be close together, he did not like any 'bits' on his plate or foods that looked 'mouldy' or 'burnt' to him. I had to try to understand the problems he had with food so I could help and encourage him to eat. I felt the issues he had about food and trying to overcome them would be an ongoing process.

When we went shopping and chose the foods he liked, he would look at each item to make sure there were no marks or damage to the packaging; if it had any, he would not want that item.

I accepted that if something did not look 'right' to him then I did not try to change his mind, because it would have been impossible!

He could not cope with things being untidy around him. He would make sure his videos and books were in a neat, straight order. When putting items in the cupboard after shopping, such as his cereal boxes, they had to be in order.

His bed linen had to be of soft material too, and if he saw any 'bits', as he would call them, all of his bed linen had to be changed. Even if it was something on a pillowcase, I couldn't just change that item, because it would cause him so much anxiety that he would not get into the bed. He could notice that something was 'wrong' with his bed linen any time during the day or night, or several times, and the linen *had* to be changed.

During his early years, I found those issues very difficult to cope with, as it caused a great deal of stress for me trying to make sure I had enough extra bed linen to cope with his unpredictable issues, when he decided the linen had to be changed.

Over the years I was learning to live around his need of a strict routine, and his problems concerning clothes, food and keeping the home as tidy as possible. I was becoming more aware of what kind of environment Jonathan felt happy in.

Not having any contact with other parents whose children had similar problems, I was trying to learn as much as I could about Jonathan's autism. I did not have any help or support or anyone to relate to. I felt it was an enormous challenge I had to deal with and try to understand, because my son's future depended on me. Many times, the whole situation overwhelmed me because I had to accept that my son was not developing as a 'normal' child. There was no future for him, and dreams I may have had for him growing up were cast aside. Our lives were a constant battle, not only with daily stressful problems, but with society too. I felt lonely not having anyone to talk over my feelings with. I knew I had to stay motivated and put on a front for society. I was able to cope with the lack of understanding about autism, and I had to be a voice for Jonathan as he had no one else to stand up for him.

I could see the progress that Jonathan was making in many ways, but I realised it was only my company he had and was used to. I needed to help him develop his social skills and be with other children. I decided to look for suitable groups that did activities he might enjoy. To my disappointment, there were no groups that took autism into consideration. There were a number of football teams for children of Jonathan's age, now approaching twelve years old, but he could not kick a ball or follow any rules to a game. It would have been impossible for him to join in. I did enquire about drama groups; again, they could not deal with autistic children, which I understood would be difficult for someone with his complex issues. My concern was for Jonathan to be able to socialise with others his own age. Having explored every group available, sadly, I had to accept that Jonathan would not be able to cope in groups and do activities that 'normal' children did at his age. Although he was making progress in most areas of his development difficulties, he was still nowhere near the stage where he could socialise, and I had to admit to myself that his peers would not accept him. This realisation hurt me very deeply. I had been working so hard to help him manage and overcome his many difficult issues, but reality showed me how much more needed to be done for Jonathan to have the same opportunities as other children. I wasn't going to give up on the idea of finding a group that Jonathan could take part in.

I needed to concentrate more on his coordination, behaviour and speech and I knew he needed to develop his social skills too. Over the past years he had needed one-to-one attention to reach the stage he was at, and I was determined that one day he would be able to join in groups with others and be accepted.

The following year I concentrated on doing more activities to improve his coordination, as well as the other skills. He did bicycle riding each week, we went to an outside tennis court regularly, not to learn to play tennis, but to improve his hand-eye coordination and feel the physical benefits. He enjoyed playing ten-pin bowling; to help his hand-eye coordination, and he was showing signs of positive improvement.

I would find as many different activities as I could for him to experience, and to find where his difficulties were with each one. My mind was focused on Jonathan being able to achieve as much as possible. Being autistic was not going to stop him.

As time passed, having been busy trying all the different activities, I was beginning to realise which ones to build on that Jonathan liked doing. Another activity I was working towards was Jonathan learning to swim. The problem that prevented it was the fact that he could not get himself changed in the changing rooms and needed support. I did not have any male friends to help him, and I could not let him go in on his own. He was making good progress at home with his bathing skills, but not enough to safely be able to cope by himself in the changing rooms.

I knew I had to wait until Jonathan was able to get himself changed, and his communication skills had improved, which was going to take time. He was still only able to express his wants or needs with sentences of two or three words.

Taking into consideration the care that Jonathan needed with his complex issues, progress was being made, although slowly. It meant my life was taken up with his care, finding new ways and ideas to keep moving forward with his development, yet the feeling of isolation was always there. Jonathan wasn't aware, as his autism prevented him from needing people around him. He was close to me, and showed affection, but was quite happy to be alone. I realised this was possibly an autistic trait. He did not want his sister too near him when she did spend time with us, which had not been a great deal over the last few years. My worries about Jonathan not having any friends brought the fears about his future into my mind, and it would start to make me feel depressed, not knowing what else to do. I had no choice but to keep working on his sensory, communication, coordination and self-care skills, with the hope that one day he would be able to go out into the community and socialise in activities that suited his needs. With the aim of Jonathan learning to swim, I enquired about swimming groups for children with autism. There were a few, but after going to look at several and talking with the group leaders, I realised the groups were large and the noise would have been too much for Jonathan to cope with. As there were only one or two helpers to support the children in the changing rooms, I decided that it was not what I wanted for Jonathan, but it gave me the idea of trying to find someone who would be willing to help. I started looking for a swimming instructor who gave one-to-one lessons, at a time that suited Jonathan.

I knew it would take time–weeks, maybe months–to find the right person I could trust, and someone Jonathan felt safe with. I decided not to rush or expect Jonathan to make a specific amount of progress in his development, to set in my mind a certain age that he needed to be learning to swim. As with everything I was helping Jonathan with, it had to be at *his* pace, and I felt confident we were not missing anything out with each learning process.

I had to accept my son was not developing as expected. I had to stop comparing him with other children, which was extremely hard to do. I felt so unhappy for him; his life seemed to be just trying to overcome daily tasks that caused him stress. He could not cope with other children or people around, and preferred to be on his own, when we were not working on his different skills. I would think to myself, 'I can help him to improve in most things, but I can't help him to socialise unless I can find a suitable group.' We were isolated in our own environment. Even though we went on various bus or train journeys, I felt all the time it was just the two of us; no one else was interested in why we were going on a short bus or train journey, and would only make comments if Jonathan got anxious or distressed about something, but no one ever offered any help. I felt utterly alone. It seemed as if I was climbing a huge mountain, not knowing if I could get to the top, or fall right back down again.

After a while, my thoughts would focus on the new idea I had about finding a swimming instructor for when Jonathan was ready to try. It bothered me a great deal how I would explain to someone about my son's autism and complex needs, and how he learns in a 'different' way. I as his mother was learning every day how to encourage him, with intended outcomes I hoped he could achieve. But to expect someone else to was going to be difficult; I decided to wait.

Always looking for different activities for Jonathan to try, I found some information about a table tennis group that met once a week. It was local and for adults and children over ten years old. I thought about table tennis, and I could visualise how it may help Jonathan with his hand-eye coordination. I spoke to the group leader, who was very pleased for us to go along and have a look. I explained to Jonathan about the table tennis club, and explained when, what time and day it would be on; which meant I had to make sure I didn't have to go out during the day, because it would have been difficult to get Jonathan to go out again for the group at six p.m.

I had to wait a few weeks, asking Jonathan each Monday, which was the day the group met, 'Do you want to go to the group?'

The day came when Jonathan said, 'Go table tennis.'

I was so pleased he wanted to try, but I was not expecting him to stay for too long. When we got to the hall where the group was held, the leader was expecting us and introduced himself and showed us the table Jonathan was going to use. One or two of the other children said hello, but Jonathan was nervous and wouldn't look at anyone. This was a trait of his autism; one I was aware would be difficult when trying to socialise. He also never wanted anyone to touch him, and he was not able to shake hands. I explained that it was a new environment and a change of routine for him, which could be difficult for him to cope with at first. The group were friendly, and I felt given time Jonathan may enjoy being there.

After the leader showed Jonathan how to bat the ball across the table a few times, he was starting to understand the concept, which was different to the tennis we played outside. When I could see the problems, Jonathan was having by batting the ball too hard and it going across the room, I asked if I could show him and explain what he needed to do. The leader and I batted the ball a few times to each other as Jonathan watched. I kept saying to Jonathan, 'Not too hard, nice and soft.' I used words he could relate to. When it was his turn with the leader, I stood by Jonathan to encourage him. After a while Jonathan had grasped the concept. I was so pleased he was learning a new skill to help his hand-eye coordination, which was my aim. I knew he would not be able to understand the rules of the game, but that didn't matter to me. He was in a different environment, with other children and adults around him, playing table tennis. His lack of communication skills was not causing him too much anxiety, as everyone just got on with their own game.

This was a big step forward in his development, and one that I could build on, so long as Jonathan wanted to go to the group. I could stay with him and encourage him, not only to play the game, but to expand on his social skills, and with time, his eye contact with people.

After the first visit to the group, Jonathan was happy to go again the following week, which he enjoyed very much. As the weeks passed, he was improving in his coordination skills and the leader suggested he might like to have another child to play a game with. I thought it was a wonderful idea when the leader introduced the other child and encouraged them to bat the ball to each other. Jonathan kept missing the ball as it was batted too fast, and was causing frustration to both of them. I asked the boy if he would slow down a little, to give Jonathan a chance to bat the ball back to him. After a few turns, Jonathan began to speed up his reactions, which was amazing to see. The leader was surprised too, by how quickly Jonathan was improving. He had the ability—the same as the others—to control the bat and ball across the table. It was a wonderful sense of achievement for us both!

We continued going to the table tennis group each week, and Jonathan was making progress with his coordination, social and communication skills. He remembered the names of members who spoke to him each week, and was gaining confidence when he said, 'hello' or 'goodbye' when leaving. He was still finding it difficult to make eye contact, but the members understood and accepted him as part of the group, which I was pleased about.

Jonathan and I played batting the ball to each other. He was speeding up his reactions as I batted the ball faster to him. As he could not understand the rules of the game, the other children didn't want to play with him. This I understood completely; they were not being unkind, they wanted to play the game properly. Jonathan was not aware of this and was quite happy with the two of us playing. I was pleased that Jonathan felt happy and included in a group that was helping him to socialise, which I had been striving to find.

As the table tennis group was on Monday evenings, this restricted us from going out during the day. I decided that was the next stage that I needed to work on. His reluctance to go anywhere and return, then make another journey later the same day caused Jonathan so much confusion and stress, and I arranged our lives around what helped him feel most at ease. I was aware that I had to try and find a way of getting him to understand that sometimes you do have to go out several times on the same day. Finding the table tennis group brought it to the front of my mind; if he was going to join other groups in the future, he had to learn to cope with doing other things during the day, as most activity groups were held in the evenings.

Routine for an autistic child is what helps them feel safe, which I understood, but I also realised that Jonathan was approaching thirteen years old and had proven he was capable of doing more. If I continued to find ways of helping him to manage the many issues, he had due to his autism, I could give him opportunities to learn and progress.

He had to try to learn to cope with change at times within his capabilities, in order to be part of the 'real world'. He needed a great deal of patience, understanding and guidance to help him work towards it, starting with predictable changes to his routine.

I had no contact with other children with autism as we were out of the 'system', so I was learning every day how my son saw 'his' world, and what helped him to cope, and adjusted our daily lives to help him feel safe and to limit his frustration.

I decided to try doing a short bus journey on Mondays, the same day he would go to the table tennis group in the evening. I spoke to Jonathan about going out in the morning, explaining that after dinner we would go to the table tennis group. As I expected, he was very reluctant to go out on the bus, because he understood it meant going out again in the evening, which he did not want to do.

When we did try the bus journey, Jonathan was very stressed and anxious wanting to go home. I kept talking to him about going out and getting home quickly, so he could go to table tennis. At first, I did not manage to go to a shop or anywhere else, because we just had to get the next bus back home, as he was so confused about why we were going out on the same day as table tennis! As I expected, he would not want to go out again, even though he was enjoying the group.

It did upset me when he chose not to go out again after a bus journey, but I knew I had to persevere with this change to his routine if I was going to be able to build on it. Several weeks went by that he did not want to go out again after a bus journey. I started doubting my reasoning for introducing change but deep down inside I knew I had to carry on with trying to encourage him to cope with it.

One Monday, I decided we wouldn't go on the bus, to see if Jonathan would go to table tennis in the evening. I did not mention the day before, as I usually did, what we were going to do the next day.

After having his breakfast and following his routine of working on his reading, numbers and clock skills, that he did every morning, he looked at the clock and said loudly, 'Bus, look, late.' Jonathan had realised the time was nine o'clock, and we would usually be walking to the bus stop to get the bus at nine fifteen. I was so shocked at his reaction and asked him if he wanted to go. He answered, 'Yes, quickly!'

We got our coats and I picked up my bag and keys, and we walked as fast as we could to the bus stop. I was expecting to have missed it, but without a minute to wait, the bus arrived. I felt so pleased that Jonathan had accepted it as part of his routine, and remembered the time of the bus to prompt *me*! I noticed after rushing to get the bus on time, he wasn't so anxious on the journey. As usual we got the next bus back home. I did not mention table tennis during the day; being happy in myself at the progress he had made that morning. We carried on with his routine of activities, and preparing for his evening meal at 5 p.m. After finishing his meal, Jonathan picked up his coat, and said, 'Table tennis.' I wasn't sure if he wanted to go, as it had been several weeks since we last attended the group. I got my things and we made our way there. I was so surprised that Jonathan had decided to go out again after the busy morning rush we had. I felt he had made progress and hoped he would enjoy going back to the group. I explained to the leader about the problems over the last few weeks and we couldn't make it; Jonathan settled back in, and soon picked up his table tennis skills again.

As time passed, our Monday bus journeys got a little easier and I was able to extend the time out of the house to complete other chores, instead of going back on the next bus straight away. Jonathan also accepted he was going out again in the evening to his group. Although it had been a difficult adjustment for him, I felt it could be built on over time and would certainly be beneficial to his development, which was always my intention and motivation as a mother: trying to do everything I could to give my son some quality of life!

Not making too many changes too soon to Jonathan's routine, we carried on with what he was used to doing. My thoughts were always on how to find different ways and opportunities to encourage Jonathan in his development. Mindful that he was thirteen years old, I felt it was time to look for a swimming instructor, to try and introduce him to swimming.

His self-care skills were improving, and his confidence in trying new things was getting better. As with everything, it all took time, and it had to be at Jonathan's pace. I contacted quite a number of swimming instructors and explained Jonathan's autism and his ability to learn. Many instructors worked with schools and groups at weekends or evenings, which were not going to suit Jonathan and his needs. To put the idea to Jonathan and get his reaction, I decided to take him to our local swimming pool to have a look and get some information. They were very helpful and understood how difficult it would be for Jonathan to join a group. They did inform me that the pool was open from 6 a.m. for adults and when I found an instructor, he would be allowed to go at that time.

After many weeks of contacting different instructors and not having any success, I decided to ask the local swimming pool staff if they would put a notice on their board for an instructor. Willing to help, they agreed to do so. A few weeks had gone by when I got a call from an instructor. I explained Jonathan's autism, hoping it would not put him off. The instructor agreed to come to the house to meet Jonathan and talk about swimming. I was pleased that he understood and wanted to take the time to get to know Jonathan a little, to see if they could get along with each other. The first meeting went well, but I was aware there needed to be several more before Jonathan and I felt comfortable about what was expected. I also needed to calculate the cost.

When we decided on the day to begin Jonathan's swimming lessons it gave me time to show him how to put on his swimming trunks and put his clothes in his bag to put into a locker, just as we saw in the changing room, reassuring him I would be by the pool watching him swim. The instructor had to encourage him to change and put his bag in the locker, and get the key which he would give to me before getting into the pool.

I was feeling very nervous, not knowing if he was coping in the changing room; when he walked out with his key with a number on it to his locker, and confidently gave it to me to hold onto. His instructor got into the pool first and encouraged Jonathan to follow. Jonathan seemed to like the water, and after a short while, was trying to swim as the instructor was guiding him. I sat watching in amazement at how well Jonathan was coping with learning to swim. I knew this was going to be wonderful progress for his development. When his first session ended and Jonathan got out of the pool to collect his locker key, I could sense his feeling of achievement. We had found another activity to help him, and one that would make use of his early mornings.

We started with one lesson a week, but after a few weeks I asked the instructor if he could do two lessons weekly, which he agreed to. I knew it would cause me financial difficulties, but as Jonathan was starting later in life to learn to swim, I wanted him to have as much time as possible to learn. I *had* to give him a chance!

Jonathan looked forward to his swimming lessons, and I could see his confidence and progress, not only in swimming, which I was happy to see, but his independent skills of getting dressed, changed and coping in the changing rooms. His instructor told me how impressed he was at Jonathan's memory, and how he followed his routine each time and did not miss anything out. This made me feel as though all the hard work over the years so far had been worthwhile, hearing from someone else, who had only known Jonathan for a short while, that they could see his ability to learn.

Realising the financial strain, it was having on me, I explained to the instructor the need to reduce Jonathan's lessons to once a week, then gradually once a fortnight, to three weeks, to allow Jonathan to get used to the adjustment of not going swimming. I didn't know how I would continue with Jonathan going swimming but somehow, I had to find a way. I knew the cost of an instructor was becoming difficult and had to end. The instructor was understanding, making sure Jonathan learnt as much as possible at each lesson so he would be able to swim by himself.

With the wonderful progress Jonathan was making learning to swim, I noticed that he preferred not to use his arms or legs to do the movements of the crawl. He liked to do breaststroke, with his feet and legs gliding under the water. The instructor had observed this too and felt Jonathan had found the best way for *him* to swim, and he would not try and change that, as he was comfortable and that was important. I agreed. I knew Jonathan's coordination problems would make it difficult for him to learn other swimming techniques, but what he had achieved so far meant he could swim safely and enjoy it, which I was happy about. The early-morning swimming activity gave me the idea to look for other things to try, whilst I tried to find another way for him to go swimming without having to pay for an instructor. I wanted Jonathan to swim regularly for the physical and mental benefits, but being vulnerable meant he needed someone to support him in the changing room.

Although swimming lessons had stopped, he still enjoyed going to the table tennis group, and accepted the routine of going out during the day, having dinner and another journey out in the evening.

Continuing to work on all his skills, progress was being made slowly. I was understanding more about how Jonathan's autism affected his daily life, and the difficulties he had. I didn't want him to stagnate in his development, so I was always thinking ahead about new activities. His behaviour was becoming more manageable as I could limit possible problems; helping Jonathan cope was my main concern.

Jonathan was approaching fourteen years old and his communication skills were very limited. Although his self-care, coordination, reading and writing skills were improving, he still only used very few words to express his needs and wants. I as his mother knew what he was saying and meant, but anyone else would find it difficult unless they got to know him, which would take a long time, if at all. His reluctance to try new foods was still an issue, one I felt would need to be worked on for the foreseeable future. I kept trying to understand his issues with food, including those related to the presentation and colours. Encouraging him to taste new foods without putting him off eating was as big a worry as his lack of speech was.

Again, thinking of the future, I wondered how he would be able to communicate. I came up with the idea of writing sentences out throughout the day and asking him to read them, then encouraging him to write sentences on what foods he liked and where he liked going. It was another way of helping Jonathan to communicate if he was not able to converse verbally. It was something I had to accept and work on. I wanted to help Jonathan become as independent as possible within his capabilities. Powered by my love, I was consumed with the determination to do everything possible within my means to help my son.

Another year had almost ended. I hadn't managed to find another new activity when swimming finished, and the table tennis group had reached a natural end when Jonathan wasn't enjoying it any longer. At fourteen years old, I knew he needed other challenges. He liked the train journeys very much and had made wonderful progress as we extended them, going to different places. Once I felt he could cope with a longer journey time, I planned a visit to a heritage train museum, which was just over an hour away. Jonathan really enjoyed the day out. I was so happy for him. I planned every detail and possible problems that we might encounter. We took our own food, pens and paper to write down things we saw, and it ended up a successful journey that gave me more ideas to build on. During our visit to the heritage train museum, where Jonathan enjoyed being able to climb onto the train to have a look, a quietly-spoken man asked me if we liked steam trains. I replied that my son was passionate about them. After enquiring about where we lived, he gave me some information about a heritage railway that was near to where we lived, and suggested we go and have a look. After thanking him, Jonathan was keen to move on to the next train in the museum. There were so many for him to explore. I began to worry about the time of our train home. I did not want to spoil the day for Jonathan, but had to explain that we could come back to the museum another day, which I intended to do in the near future. We had a pleasant journey home, and I thought about the progress Jonathan had made during our visit to the museum. He coped better than I expected in the new environment. When we went to look at the menu in the café, the different smells of food were not affecting him. I knew he wouldn't want anything to eat or drink, but showing him the café and menu, suggesting that when we made another visit, he could have lunch there. It was an opportunity to build on to help him progress in his development.

I made contact with the local heritage railway and found out that they ran steam trains every Saturday and Sunday for the public. I was so pleased to have found another new interest that would encourage Jonathan to go out of the house and into a different environment.

After making our first visit to the heritage railway and having had several rides on the steam strains, Jonathan was happy and interested at looking at the different trains. He coped with the noise of the trains and looked happily around the station and at a stall that sold used books and videos. To my surprise, Jonathan picked up a steam train video that interested him. I asked him if he would like to buy it and watch it at home, to which he replied, 'Watch.' They were a reasonable cost, and I thought it may help him develop his new interest.

Having made several visits to the heritage railway—which Jonathan looked forward to-the people who worked there began to recognise us, and were very friendly towards Jonathan, which was an unexpected change. After getting to know the people and feeling at ease, I was able to engage in conversation about trains. I had limited opportunities to talk with others. I knew Jonathan felt happy there, and it was helping us both to socialise. On one particular visit, a guard who always made a point of saying hello, and asking Jonathan if he was enjoying his train rides. He mentioned that the railway relied on volunteers to do many different jobs to help raise funds for track work and restoring trains. They have used items stalls, and a café where volunteers are needed. The qualified train drivers gave their time voluntary at weekends for the heritage railway to open to the public.

I explained our circumstances, and of Jonathan's autism, and he reassured me they welcomed anyone, and we would be shown what needed to be done and could then choose what tasks suited us.

I felt it would be beneficial for Jonathan, not being in school, and would give him the opportunity to volunteer on weekdays and have a train ride at weekends.

I agreed to go along on the arranged day and time to find out more about how the railway worked. On our first visit, we were shown around the work shed, where the trains were repaired, painted and cleaned for public use on running days. Whilst walking round the work shed, I was observing Jonathan's reactions to the different sounds of tools being used. We would be supervised by an experienced member of staff for safety reasons if we did any job in the work shed. At that time, I didn't feel Jonathan would be able to stay in that environment, with the different noises and the dust all around. The person showing us round said we would be given overalls and ear protectors to wear. After our tour of the work shed, I asked if there were other jobs to be done outside and was informed that the railway was planning to start a project in the near future. I explained that I would like Jonathan to learn to use different tools if possible, and enquired if it was legal for him to be in the work shed at fourteen years old. The railway agreed to let Jonathan on the premises as long as I was with him at all times, which I intended to be. I asked Jonathan if he wanted to come back to the work shed and he said yes. I felt that being in a real working environment that interested him was going to give him the opportunity to learn new skills.

On our way home, I spoke to Jonathan about going to work in the shed, about wearing overalls and gloves, so we wouldn't get dirty, and ear protectors to stop the noise of the different tools. He was anxious about getting dirty, and the noise. I reassured him there were lots of other things to do.

The day came for us to go to the heritage railway work shed. When we arrived, we were introduced to the other volunteers and given some gloves, overalls and ear protectors. The leader asked if he would like to look at a large steam crane that they used for lifting up track. Jonathan was keen to have a look and walked confidently beside the leader. I followed behind, observing Jonathan's reactions, which were amazingly positive.

When we got to the crane, the leader explained that the railway was in the process of restoring it, which was going to take quite a long time as it was the volunteers who spent time each week scraping the rust off before any painting could be done. We were asked to carry on scraping off as much rust as possible with the tools we were given. After being shown how to use the scraping tools, Jonathan put on his overalls, gloves and goggles, and started scraping at the rust. On seeing how enthusiastic he was, I thought I had to try too. After a while, we were managing to scrape a lot off. The leader felt we were coping and decided to go and get me a drink of tea, and water for Jonathan. I could see the concentration on Jonathan's face, scraping away at this huge crane, that I didn't think would ever be restored. I began to feel we were doing a 'useful' job, and in a friendly environment. After two hours of scraping the rust, and Jonathan not stopping, it was time to put everything away and wash our hands, ready to go home for lunch. I did explain to the leader that we would only be able to stay for a short while to begin with until Jonathan got used to it, as his mealtime routine was important to him.

Having enjoyed being in the work shed and doing a 'real' job, I knew it was going to be the opportunity that would help Jonathan's confidence, coordination and communication skills over time. He looked forward to his weekly visits to the work shed, and had the ability to understand that the work being done on the crane and trains would enable them to be used on the track when finished. At home he would draw trains, which was wonderful progress. I encouraged him to write words to describe his pictures.

Although I was still concerned about his limited speech, I was amazed at the way he was taking to his work on the crane and thinking about it more when drawing different pictures.

The other volunteers could see how much Jonathan was progressing, and managing the scraping that most people would lose interest in after a short time.

The leader asked if Jonathan would like to be shown how to use a tool that would get the rust off a little faster. It was a noisy tool and ear protectors, goggles and gloves had to be worn, and it could only be used for ten minutes before you had to have a break. After having it demonstrated to us, I decided to use it first, so I could understand the effects, and how to explain it to Jonathan. After using it for five minutes, I thought it may be a difficult tool to get used to, as the vibration felt in the hands might prove unpleasant for Jonathan. Having got his protective goggles, gloves and ear protectors on, the leader was helping him hold the tool, which was called a needle gun. I watched very closely to make sure Jonathan was holding it properly. Within a few minutes of starting the tool and seeing how much rust was coming off the crane, I was expecting Jonathan to want to stop. The leader was carefully supervising and ready to turn it off after ten minutes, which he did. We were waiting for Jonathan's reaction when he took his ear protectors off. I asked him if he liked using the gun and showed him how much rust he took off. Jonathan said, 'More needle gun,' and went to put on his ear protectors again. The leader and

I explained there would be no more until next week. We were pleased and surprised by how he controlled it, and how he was not frightened by the vibration or dull banging sound through the ear protectors. We carried on scraping with the tools that we first used, and Jonathan accepted that he could only use the needle gun for a short time.

That morning Jonathan had learnt to use a heavy mechanical tool with great care and concentration and could see the results of his work. He was learning about the safety of using different tools, and what was dangerous. Experiencing a real working environment that interested him, Jonathan was learning and remembering everything, and confirming to me that there was so much more for him to achieve by giving him as many opportunities as possible.

I was so excited about Jonathan's voluntary work, I wanted to inform Kelly, whom we hadn't seen for a long time. I thought it may encourage her to get involved with Jonathan after learning of his progress and new interest. Sadly, no effort was made to find out how Jonathan enjoyed his 'work,' by his sister or father.

Our weekly visits to the work shed were becoming very interesting, and Jonathan was eager to do whatever tasks were required, as well as carrying on with getting the rust off the crane, using the needle gun for a short time. I could see how he was understanding the sense of responsibility and how every task had to be done right. Once shown how to do a task, Jonathan remembered it in detail. He got the opportunity to learn how to use a number of different tools; some were electrical, some mechanical, and he could remember what tools were needed for a certain task. I was absolutely amazed how Jonathan was settling into the environment and the skills he was learning. I realised, if he had been in a school, he would have missed out on the wonderful opportunity that he was now experiencing.

The volunteers were all friendly and helpful towards Jonathan and me. One volunteer, who recognised Jonathan's need to finish at a certain time to go home for his lunch, suggested we go to the work shed earlier to give Jonathan more time to learn different skills. As he usually got there earlier than the others, he could help Jonathan with his tasks.

I thought it was a really good idea, as Jonathan got up early anyway. It would mean leaving the house sooner and not giving him time to watch his videos. I had been trying to find a way of distracting him from doing that but couldn't. Now, this suggestion of Jonathan going to 'work' early was the incentive to achieve that outcome, even if it was only once a week. Jonathan accepted the idea without hesitation, and we started our voluntary work early each week, without him worrying about not finishing in time before going home for his lunch. I did suggest to him after a number of weeks that he take his lunch and eat it at the work shed café room; he rejected that idea, which I accepted.

One particular early morning start at the railway, the volunteer who usually got there before us was late, and we were waiting outside the gates for some time, not knowing if he was going to turn up. It surprised me that Jonathan was willing to wait. The volunteer finally turned up and apologised for the delay. He opened the gates and work shed. He then said he had missed his breakfast, and would be cooking himself a sausage sandwich in the kitchen before starting work. Having made me a cup of tea and got Jonathan a drink of water, he asked if we would like a sandwich. I looked at Jonathan, as he had heard the word sausage, and asked if he wanted to try a sandwich. To my amazement, he said, 'Yes please!' Both the volunteer and I could not believe his response, and he began cooking the sausages. After getting his overalls on and sorting out his gloves and goggles, the sandwich was ready. I watched how Jonathan enjoyed it, thinking he must be hungry, having had his cereal at 5 a.m., or maybe it was because he felt different in a working environment. I was pleased he had eaten something because of the energy he needed for the next few hours. I couldn't help feeling what tremendous progress Jonathan was making by being given this opportunity!

After finishing another morning working on the steam crane, I had to remind Jonathan it was time to go for lunch. I think he may have stayed longer, as he was so engrossed in his work. The leader asked whether we would like to come for another morning during the week, as Jonathan was enjoying it so much. Being early was not a problem, as the volunteer who regularly did so commented how he wanted to help Jonathan do other jobs, and it would give him the time to show him more skills. I thanked him for his kindness, something we had not experienced in society before now, and agreed to another day. Going two mornings a week and having to leave the house early, Jonathan became less obsessed with watching his videos, and I felt that going to the work shed was having beneficial outcomes for him.

He continued to concentrate on scraping the rust off the steam crane and seemed determined to finish it. It surprised everyone how much he had done each week, and the leader decided to give the task to Jonathan. In one way I was pleased that he was given responsibility and trusted to do the job, but also, I felt that it may be an impossible task to expect of him.

As time passed, most of the rust had been scraped off, and Jonathan could see and sense his achievement. When he had completed scraping the whole crane, all the members came to have a look and praised Jonathan for his good work.

Then it had to be painted! I felt so proud of Jonathan and his achievement, and knew he would finish painting the whole crane, however long it took, as no one else had got as far as Jonathan with scraping the rust off.

Being able to relate to real trains and cranes by working in that environment, Jonathan was 'growing up.'

Although he had communication, sensory, and coordination issues, he had something where he could be himself, and achieve skills that may never have been recognised, had he not been given the opportunity to try.

Jonathan's life was structured; doing his reading, writing, numbers and his clock skills, working on his self-care and sensory issues, progress was being made. Having his work, as he began to relate to it as, was giving him the incentive to go out of the house the weekdays and weekends, which he didn't do before finding the heritage railway. It was a place he enjoyed and felt safe in; it was giving him the opportunity to learn a variety of skills, along with his social and communication skills, which I considered to be as important too. Jonathan was learning and being encouraged to make eye contact with other people and greeting everyone by shaking their hand. These social skills that are taken for granted by most people are difficult issues for children with autism, and need to be continually encouraged. It was also helping me be able to talk with people—not just about trains, although that was the main topic. One or two of the volunteers were interested in Jonathan, which pleased me, because I was able to talk about his autism, and all the other things he does at home. I felt in a way, it was helping them understand autism, and hopefully would encourage them to continue to include anyone who is interested in railways and was able to do any voluntary work.

I felt Jonathan had got over another hurdle in his development and had come a long way since that fear of him being institutionalised by the age of ten or eleven. Now, at fourteen years old, he was experiencing opportunities that I felt would have positive outcomes for him in the future. It was these thoughts that made me determined to give Jonathan every possible chance in life, to let him develop and express himself to be who he wanted to be, and being labelled autistic was not going to stop him!

Sadly, his sister and father chose not to be part of Jonathan's progress, after many attempts to include them.

Over the following months we continued going to the work shed two mornings a week and for a train ride at weekends. Jonathan was learning to use different tools which he liked: hammers, spanners of all sizes to undo rusty bolts, which there were many on the steam crane. Also, from time to time, he would have a sandwich that the volunteer prepared in the mornings; it was always sausages, and he got used to cooking it the way Jonathan liked. I was so pleased he was eating something more substantial than cereal, because he used a lot of energy doing his work. Getting used to eating a warm sandwich helped during the dark cold mornings when Jonathan would still want to go to 'work'. I admired and respected his determination to finish the crane; it was more than his need to keep to his routine; and that is what motivated me.

The end of the year was approaching, and the volunteers explained that the work shed and trains were decorated for Christmas. They said we could help to put Santa faces and *Thomas the Tank Engine* faces on the trains, which the children liked. I explained that Jonathan wouldn't want to do that, as he had grown out of children's things and would not understand why the work shed was decorated for Christmas. I asked Jonathan if he wanted to help and the answer was, 'No, for little children!' It meant we had to miss going to the work shed during December, but we offered to come in after Christmas to tidy everything away, which I felt would be more helpful for Jonathan, as he still found Christmas difficult.

He enjoyed his 'work' and accepted that the heritage railway was decorated at Christmas for children. He knew that he was going to help to clear it all away when it was finished. It helped him cope, and it was another opportunity for Jonathan to learn and progress. It was the end of the year, and he was looking forward to starting his 'work' again in the new year.

Chapter Four Fifteen to Twenty Years Old

Over the weeks that we didn't go to the work shed, we continued with all the skills that Jonathan had been learning and continued our early morning walks to McDonald's. The weather was cold, it being December, and Jonathan was now comfortable with the idea of sitting inside to eat toast. I was so pleased about it, even though it had taken a long time for him to feel confident about doing so. On our walk to McDonalds, we saw houses decorated for Christmas with different coloured lights, and gardens with Christmas novelty scenes, which helped Jonathan to cope with the season. I talked about Christmas and presents. He wasn't overjoyed with it, but understood that it would be finished soon and everything would go back to normal.

We also made a few short train journeys. I wanted to see how Jonathan would cope. After planning our journey, I intended to visit a shop which sold videos that might interest him. I was trying to guide Jonathan to feel part of the Christmas season. He would see that the station had a Christmas tree and decorations and that shops we passed were decorated with brightly coloured lights and Christmas scenes. I was aware of more people being around us but I kept talking to him and encouraging him to look at the different decorations.

When we got to the shop that sold videos, I would encourage Jonathan to look at the variety of them. I did not expect him to take much interest, but I tried to help him cope in that environment. To my surprise, after a few such journeys Jonathan felt happy about going on the short train trips, and knew what to expect in the shop he was going to visit.

This was wonderful progress! He was managing to be part of the Christmas season. He began to enjoy going to buy a video. The train on the way home was busy during the Christmas weeks; at times we chose to stand in the corridor to look out of the window. This took his mind off all the people around him and gave us different things to look at and talk about. It also helped me to feel a little more excited about Christmas. I knew I wouldn't be seeing Kelly, which hurt me deeply. I wanted Jonathan not to get too anxious and stressed about Christmas; to enjoy it in his own way. I felt Jonathan was changing the way in which he was understanding Christmas.

Having the wonderful opportunity to work at the heritage railway was helping him to cope with the Christmas season.

After Christmas, Jonathan was looking forward to going back to the work shed. He had helped to put away the decorations, and saw the work shed return to the environment he was used to working in. Jonathan was looking forward to starting work on the crane. I too was looking forward to be going to the work shed. Being within a friendly environment, it gave me the opportunity to talk to someone. I had spent a lot of time on my own. I was with Jonathan, but I felt mentally lonely. Doing the voluntary work helped me to feel part of something, which had positive and beneficial effects for us both.

A new year had begun, and I was happy for Jonathan that he had an interest which he felt settled in. I could visualise all the different tasks he would have the opportunity to experience at the heritage railway; this would help him in his development.

Meanwhile, my thoughts about the relationship with Kelly were hurting me very much. She didn't make any effort to come and see me or Jonathan over Christmas; we hadn't seen much of her for many months. I felt as a mother my daughter would never want me to be part of her life. She was being influenced to feel that I was rejecting her for Jonathan but this was so far from the truth. I was in an extremely difficult situation. I had no support but I always tried to include Kelly in Jonathan's life, to show her the progress he was making.

It felt as though Kelly and her father did not believe me and thought that Jonathan could not be capable of such progress. There was nothing more I could do. I had to keep encouraging and helping Jonathan in his development, which I felt was the right thing to do, even if my daughter was rejecting me for doing something that she and her father did not consider worthwhile.

The day arrived when Jonathan and I were starting 'work' again at the heritage railway. It was a cold January morning. Jonathan was looking forward to going back, which I was pleased about too. It motivated me to go; the cold weather wasn't going to put me off! When we arrived, the volunteer, who usually arrived there early, turned on a few heaters to warm the work shed a little. He was expecting us! He had prepared the tools for the tasks that were needed that day and had already started cooking some sausages for a sandwich.

Although, the work shed was cold, the heaters were on and with the smell of sausages cooking, Jonathan was able to settle back into the environment. He accepted the offer of a warm sandwich before starting his work.

All the decorations had been taken down; it was back to a normal work shed. Jonathan saw and liked it! With the crane scraped clear of rust, it was ready to be undercoated with paint especially for that task. It was going to take a number of weeks to undercoat the whole crane but Jonathan could understand and accept it, as he was choosing how much he was going to do on each day of work on it. He didn't rush with the painting, which was carefully and neatly applied. I saw how he was concentrating on the way he would start painting and deciding in his own mind where he would finish until the next time. The other volunteers could see how engrossed he was and therefore wouldn't interrupt him by talking to him, realising that he was enjoying doing it on his own, within a friendly environment.

Seeing Jonathan progress in the work shed was helping me to understand him further and how he saw his 'work'. He had to complete a task in a way that he wanted to. There was no rushing him; he would always do it neatly and properly, however long it took. Most of the jobs in the work shed did take time to finish. Jonathan just wanted to do his work; he didn't need to socialise, which I felt was part of his autism, although he always said hello to the volunteers. That was all he wanted to do. His limited communication skills prevented him from talking about his interest in trains. I always tried to help him say to the other volunteers a few words about what he was doing on the crane, to encourage his social skills. Thankfully, everyone accepted and understood his autism and could see how much effort he put into his work. I was hoping that, with time, Jonathan's communication skills would continue to improve.

We continued to work on his reading, speech, writing, sensory, coordination and self-care skills. His diet was varying a little more but getting him to try different foods was an ongoing issue with him!

I felt I was doing the best that I could to help Jonathan have some quality of life whilst continuing to develop his progression.

Although working at the heritage railway was giving him the opportunity to learn new skills and use his energy to exert any pent-up emotions he had, I was aware that Jonathan was becoming frustrated with himself because he couldn't verbally express his wants or needs. He got quite stressed at times and although I knew most of the time that which he meant, I had to admit to myself as a mother that Jonathan was finding it difficult to cope in situations where people couldn't understand him, and needed me to explain what he meant.

Approaching fifteen years old; I continued to worry about his future. With the progress he was making in all his other skills his communication and speech were still limited. He really enjoyed his work at the heritage railway and it was a wonderful opportunity for him, but I knew he was becoming frustrated within himself. Unsure of what else I could do, I tried to keep him busy and mentally active. Worry about his future began to consume my thoughts and depress me. When I thought about how well my daughter Kelly was doing, at only a few years older than Jonathan, I began doubting my ability as a mother and just what I was trying to achieve. I had no contact with other parents of autistic children; I was having to learn every day how to understand my son and how I could help him. Trying to find ways to teach him, to develop his skills; I devoted all my efforts and strength to the point of exhaustion but I hadn't yet found a way to help his communication skills. I began to feel like a failure.

My daughter had decided she now did not want anything to do with me. She wrote me a letter to say that she felt I left her out just to have Jonathan to myself. That is how she saw it and felt. It upset me very much! My hopes and plan were for us all to work together for Jonathan's future. As a parent, I admitted I did not know all the answers on looking after an autistic child. I had no experience of autism. All I knew was that I had to help my son, whatever it took. I thought that maybe when my daughter was older, she may come to understand. For now, I had to accept her rejection.

As the heritage railway was not running weekend trains over the winter months, going to the work shed during the week was helping Jonathan focus on painting the crane; and understanding the train rides would begin again soon. It was another learning opportunity for him, just as he had to accept at Christmas the work shed and trains were decorated for the children's sake, which he felt was 'not for him'. He was growing up and changing in a positive way, with him making his own decisions.

Having got used to going for a train ride at weekends, while waiting for them to begin again, I wanted to keep up with the idea of going out on a Saturday or Sunday and not fall back into the ritual of not going out because his usual place of interest was not open. I was aware how easy it would be to stagnate so I decided to try a longer bus journey or train journeys to a different town on alternate weekends. Again, I had to plan every detail and consider possible problems.

He had coped over the Christmas weeks on the short train journeys to the railway museum—which I was planning to visit again when it opened—and it gave me the idea to expand on them. Other ideas were to visit a castle that we had been to, or indoor museums that had train memorabilia, along with aeroplane and car museums; trying to show Jonathan other types of transport. It would also give him ideas to draw and write sentences about; different words to learn to read and speak. I was always trying to make every new experience an opportunity to learn, and to understand Jonathan's way of seeing *his* world. I would find out that other interests he might have that I could expand on.

Many of the visits to castles or museums were not successful but I felt that trying them was helping me to understand his autism and how it affected him. That was my aim! I came to realise that trains were his main interest, which helped me to accept and understand. Castles and museums did not really interest him, because as I understood his autism, he could not relate them to his life, whereas trains he could; they were real to him. Jonathan had no imagination.

It is very difficult for someone like Jonathan, who can only understand time as now, or perhaps a day or so ahead. This is why routine is so important to him, and any change must be made gradually.

At the work shed, Jonathan had almost finished painting the undercoat on the crane, and the leader along with the other volunteers were very pleased with his progress. As Easter was approaching and the train rides were due to begin for the public, Jonathan felt pleased with himself. I could sense his achievement over seeing it nearly completed with the first coat of paint applied. The leader was talking about displaying the crane during the summer at an open day event for the public, once it had been painted black. As it was only a few months away, I couldn't be sure that Jonathan would complete it in time, but I talked about it to him and explained that I could help, to which he answered, 'No, Jonathan do it.' This was *his* target to paint the crane by the summer, and to see it moving on the track. I felt so proud of him and his sense of responsibility despite all his problems.

As each week went by Jonathan concentrated on painting the crane black. It was clear for him to see if he had missed any undercoat because it was grey, and he would make sure every corner or gap was painted. He did not stop for at least three hours at a time. It was a task that may have seemed tedious to anyone else but to Jonathan, it was a project he wanted to do and to finish, and to see it working on the track.

It was a task *he* had completed. Having shown his ability to the other volunteers, I was so grateful that Jonathan had the opportunity to prove that being autistic does not mean not to achieve; people with autism just need to be given a chance!

As the weeks went by Jonathan was near to finishing painting the crane. The train rides for the public had begun for Easter; this meant Jonathan could look forward to going out at weekends to visit the railway, and not to just work in the shed. We knew the drivers and guards on the trains and they were always friendly towards Jonathan and me. It was an environment Jonathan felt happy and safe in. He could be himself.

I felt I was doing all I could for him at the time but was still searching for new ideas to expand his development. With not being able to go swimming, and table tennis having finished, I knew I could not stagnate. The railway work was a wonderful experience for Jonathan. This motivated me to find other interests to help him. Knowing his ability, I had to keep finding other opportunities for him.

I continued to work on his sensory, coordination, communication, reading, and self-care skills, which I knew was an ongoing way of helping Jonathan, and progress was being made. With his amazing ability to remember, I realised he had a photographic memory; whenever I was showing him how to do a new task, it had to be done step by step, and correctly, because he would remember the instructions and any changes afterwards would be difficult for him to accept. I found this ability fascinating and connected it to his autism.

He had the ability to remember journeys, and which way to go by car, rail or bus. It gave me ideas on how I could use these skills when planning journeys.

I purchased an atlas and started pointing out all the places we had been to by train, car or on the bus. I would get him to write them down and say the place names, write sentences about them, draw a picture of what he could connect each place with. I encouraged him to find the heritage railway museum that we'd gone to on the map, and the railway he 'worked' at. He was showing me how he could remember each place he saw. I knew this skill could be developed further. I wanted to visit other railways to expand his development.

We continued going to the work shed and having a train ride at weekends until the crane was finished. When Jonathan finally finished painting the crane, the leader and other volunteers were surprised and pleased with his progress. We were looking forward to seeing it working out on the track, when the date was arranged. Jonathan felt happy with his achievement and was looking forward to seeing it working. After that, I knew it was time for us to visit other heritage railways at weekends that I had found the details of.

Having watched the steam crane working outside on the track, I felt so proud of Jonathan's achievements. People who had turned up for the open day were commenting on how good it looked! I was talking to Jonathan about the wonderful job he had done and how the people liked it. Several people asked about the crane, which gave me the opportunity to say that Jonathan, who is autistic, painted it. They congratulated him on his work, which made Jonathan feel that he had achieved something. When we went to the work shed the following week, the leader said they wanted to start on the new project, and wondered if Jonathan would like to help.

He showed us outside the work shed an area which the railway group were planning to develop into a narrow-gauge train and track. The trains were smaller and the track would be going a short distance around the back of the work shed. The public would be able to ride on some of the old carriages that used to take miners to the coalmine many years ago.

The heritage railway was hoping to set up a small museum to show people about the history of narrow-gauge trains once used by miners in the area. I thought it was a wonderful project to be part of, even though I had no idea how or when it would be finished. All I could see was an old shed, rusty carriages, and pieces of track. The ground was neither flat nor level, and there were stones and rubble everywhere. The leader explained the ground needed to be dug to level it. There were other volunteers working on the project during the week too. We looked at the shed where we could make a drink or sandwich, and the tool shed. I wasn't sure if Jonathan would like the change from working inside the shed to being outside but all I could do was encourage him and talk about the new track and trains he could take a ride on when it was finished. The volunteer who was overseeing the project explained the different tasks that needed to be done, one step at a time. He was very understanding of Jonathan and appreciated that Jonathan knew much more about railways than he could verbally express. He spent time showing Jonathan the pieces of track which were already laid down leading to the shed with a smaller train in it, which was being restored. By having some track put down first it meant that the narrow-gauge train could be pushed in and out of the shed in order to be worked on.

He showed Jonathan how to tighten the fish bolts (as they were called), on the track before pushing the train out. Using a large spanner, after being shown what to do, Jonathan carefully made sure that the bolts were tight. He understood the train would de-rail if they weren't. The volunteer was very pleased that Jonathan understood and learnt very quickly what was needed. He showed us the area which was required for digging over for levelling. I knew this was going to be quite strenuous and would take a long time but the railway group were not in a hurry, and appreciated the volunteers were giving up their time to do whatever they could.

Jonathan started digging the area he was shown. It was difficult manual work and I was worried that he would not have sufficient energy. I asked if I could bring in some food to cook for him whilst he was digging. The volunteer in charge thought that this was a good idea and showed me how to use the basic cooking facilities in the shed.

After a few weeks Jonathan was enjoying the digging; having a rest by coming into the shed for a sandwich, then choosing to go back to his work for a while. As I went outside several times to make sure he was alright, I knew he wanted to just get on with his job. He was able to use as much energy, and at times get rid of his frustration by doing a physical task. He was also showing me that he was progressing in his development, and capable of understanding how the project would be finished. The volunteer would explain to Jonathan and me where the track was going to go for the train rides, and the old carriages which would require painting. There were so many different tasks for Jonathan to try and I knew he was enjoying being part of the project.

As we went to 'work' those early mornings, there were only three of us with the volunteer in charge of the project. It was wonderfully quiet working outside. I did jobs like sorting out the shed and tool shed which I felt were helpful. Jonathan seemed content and happy being at the railway.

I started making plans to visit other heritage railways at weekends, to expand his experience and to encourage him to use his skills at remembering, by helping to plan a route, which involved a number of issues which had to be taken into consideration. I felt his ability to remember details needed to be encouraged and developed.

I found it difficult to understand that part of his autism. He was not able to verbally communicate as a 'normal' person approaching sixteen years old, and yet he had these amazing skills and a photographic memory! It continued to show me that children with autism were so undervalued in society, because they are not understood. I wanted to keep learning and developing Jonathan's skills in every way I could.

The day arrived when we were going to visit a new heritage railway. It would involve boarding two trains, there and back. The first part of the journey he was familiar with, then we had to walk to another station to get the next train to the heritage railway. Both parts of the journey were short, which were planned to enable us to get home quickly if needed. When we reached the new heritage railway, Jonathan was very interested in looking around the work sheds that we were able to do, and to see other trains being restored. There were trains running for the public to ride on, as it was a working, repairing and restoring railway. It was very interesting, and the people were friendly towards us.

Seeing how interested Jonathan was, one of the workmen asked if Jonathan wanted to climb onto a train to have a look at the controls. He was very happy to do that. Having spent quite a long time exploring the work sheds and getting onto a number of different trains, I knew his hobby and interest of trains was going to continue to develop and help him to progress in a variety of skills, and mature.

At the back of my mind, the worry about his future was always there. Although he had proven that fear of being institutionalised wrong, I knew he had many issues that may never improve enough for him to live an independent life; something every parent of a child who has a disability constantly worries about. All the amazing skills Jonathan had, did not mean he could live the life, or have the same opportunities as someone 'normal' has, but all I could do was try as much as possible to build a life that Jonathan felt happy and safe with, which was the most important thing I could do. As a mother, I had accepted he wouldn't have a job or career, marriage or children or friends. It hurt me deeply, but I had to accept reality so I could concentrate on my aims for him.

My life was consumed with caring for my son and holding onto the hope that progress would continue, and his speech would improve.

His self-care skills were improving as time went on, but health issues like dental care and physical checks with a doctor were extremely difficult to deal with. His fear and dislike of hospitals and doctors made it a concern and worry for me. I had to be aware of any change in his health or behaviour because he couldn't verbally tell me. Being a single parent with no support, the responsibility was overwhelming. If he had a cold or was not feeling well, I had to find out why. Our experience with doctors was not pleasant, as little interest was shown, I felt, because he was autistic.

I decided to find a dentist privately; one who would take the time with Jonathan, however difficult he was at the start. We visited a few and after getting Jonathan's reaction, very often it meant leaving before any checks on his teeth could be done. I felt the atmosphere the same as Jonathan did as soon as we went into a dentist, and I knew if it was not the right one for Jonathan, I would apologise and we would leave. I did not want him to have a fear of going to a dentist. I knew however that if I could find the right person, he would be willing to go. After phoning and seeing a number of dentists, I finally managed to find one that was considerate and understanding. Having booked an early first appointment, Jonathan was anxious, but I kept reassuring him that everything would be alright, and I would be with him. When the dentist called him in, he was calm and pleasant, talking to Jonathan and showing him pictures of teeth. He asked if he could look in his mouth and make sure that his teeth were healthy. The dentist used words which I had explained that Jonathan would understand.

The visit went well. The dentist was pleased with his teeth. We booked another appointment for six weeks ahead. I wanted to build up the trust between Jonathan and the dentist, despite the financial strain on myself. To ensure Jonathan did not have a fear of dentists, it was important that time and care was given to him at each visit.

Trying to understand my son's autism and how it affected every aspect of his life was at times an impossible, frustrating and heartbreaking experience.

I had to keep finding ways to help him develop and progress. As he couldn't express himself verbally, he would become stressed and angry if he wasn't understood. His emotional and mental health were affected, and I tried to understand his frustration. When he was disappointed about something he would withdraw into himself, and not let me comfort him. If he didn't feel himself, he would go quiet and want to be alone.

I had to be aware of all his emotions at all times as he couldn't explain just how he was feeling. That is why finding the right dentist was important for Jonathan; he interpreted a person's voice if it was too harsh, or had an unfriendly attitude. On occasions when we had to visit a doctor, the doctor would talk over Jonathan as if he didn't matter, or couldn't understand. This made Jonathan react in a stressful manner. The doctor would offer drugs to 'calm' him down! That kind of attitude made me angry and I wondered why I bothered to bring him, when they were not interested in finding out what the problem is.

Society did not understand or care enough to understand autism or the effects it had on a person. Society was too quick to judge an autistic person's behaviour as 'out of control' and that they needed drugs to calm them down.

My son was sensitive to different environments, people, their tone of voice, and attitude towards him. I realised that was Jonathan's way of expressing his feelings in situations he didn't feel safe in. It was an autistic trait that was important and needed to be recognised! Whenever Jonathan had a reaction to a certain person, I understood why and knew how he was feeling. I respected his judgement and would move him away from the person or situation before it caused him more anxiety. It became a 'sixth sense', that I accepted he had. I respected his feelings at all times, however difficult it seemed. I knew if the right people were around him, and in situations where he felt safe, then that was going to be my guidance to help build a life where he felt happy and safe, and able to be himself.

We continued to work at the heritage railway on the narrow-gauge project and visited different ones at weekends to expand his experience. Jonathan was enjoying the work on the narrow-gauge and liked digging and levelling off the ground for the track. He was settled in that environment, developing a maturity.

He liked planning visits to different railways and finding them on the map. We talked about how we would get there, train times, how we'd take our own food. After visiting a railway, he would draw pictures of it and I would encourage him to write a sentence using words he understood. His ability to draw trains in detail amazed me! He was drawing straight lines freehand and could remember the name and number of each train he saw. His sense of direction and interest in road signs gave me ideas on how to expand these skills. His verbal communication skills were limited, even though he had an amazing memory which he showed in his drawings. I intended to encourage with drawing as a way of communicating. I was accepting that speech may always be difficult for him, but at least there was another way of communicating.

As the heritage railway was preparing for the next Christmas season, it meant Jonathan could not ride on the trains. We were working on the project outside so we did not have to stop as we had when working inside the work shed when it had to be decorated for Christmas. This helped Jonathan because he could keep to his routine and not have his 'work' area disrupted. Although it was cold outside, he appreciated coming into the shed for a warm sandwich and a rest. It was his place of work! I respected his motivation to want to keep going to the railway even when it was raining and cold. Very little work could be done there at times, but he had to go and try to do *something*. I was so pleased with his sense of responsibility that it inspired me to go and try to achieve something of good use, for whatever time we spent there during the winter months.

As Jonathan was approaching seventeen years old, I felt he was doing an extremely valuable job. The work experience he was gaining, although voluntary, was giving him opportunities to develop and expand his skills that he would not have been given if he had been in a 'special school'. I knew as a seventeen-year-old, despite all of his problems, Jonathan was proving just what a responsible, hard-working person he was. In the right environment, and given the opportunities, autism can be channelled into areas of interest to the person, with amazing outcomes.

When the heritage railways were preparing for Christmas, Jonathan was quite happy to go on a train or bus journey to visit a shop which sold videos. He knew what to expect and was coping with the Christmas season more. I felt that he was making more progress, coping in that environment of more people, sounds, music, smells of different foods. I still carried bottles of oils with me for him to smell if things got too much for him; I was appreciating how important and helpful aromatherapy oils were for Jonathan. He was enjoying Christmas a little more, and looking forward to going to the video shop, and we managed to visit a book shop. This was wonderful progress!

It had been many years of not being able to like the Christmas season, and now to see Jonathan able to enjoy it in his own way made me feel so much happier for him.

My thoughts turned to his father and sister. If only they would take an interest in his life, they would see the amazing progress Jonathan was making. I knew that was not going to happen; Jonathan and I would enjoy Christmas in our own way.

When Christmas was over, we talked about going back to 'work' at the heritage railway. He was happy at the prospect of going to work on the narrow-gauge project, which would take a number of years to complete. I felt I needed to look for other opportunities to give him a variety of activities, although trains were his favourite interest. I accepted, but I did not want to stagnate.

Thinking about his skills with remembering directions, places and signs, I had an idea about trying a different form of transport to see if he would be interested. The idea of going on a canal boat came to me, as we lived near a mooring and I saw a sign for canal boats to hire for a day. I was always looking to introduce Jonathan to different things and decided to make enquiries about hiring a canal boat for a few hours, and find out about the costs and what was involved, as, I had never been on one before.

I talked to Jonathan about canals, got pictures of boats and showed him on a map where they were. He seemed very interested, which I was pleased about, but I was worried about not being able to manage it now that I'd put the idea to him. I wanted to give him the opportunity to try.

When the spring came, I made the arrangement to hire a small boat. I would be given instruction and the canal was not busy at that time of year.

When the day arrived for us to go on the boat—which was at a very reasonable cost, having explained my situation and reasons—I tried not to show Jonathan how nervous I was! After being shown how to steer the small boat, Jonathan was happy to go for a short ride along the canal. I was amazed how easy it was to steer, and Jonathan seemed happy to be experiencing a completely different form of transport. After a while of steering, I asked Jonathan if he wanted to try, which he was very eager to do. I could not believe how careful he was at steering and keeping the boat straight. He was so much better than I was. I felt so happy for him because he was proving what amazing ability he had. It also confirmed for me that his hand-eye coordination had improved over the years; this gave me hope that other issues would improve too.

Our first canal boat experience went very well, and I realised that Jonathan had found another interest which would give him different opportunities to learn new skills, in an environment that was pleasant and calming for him.

I continued encouraging him with his reading, writing and drawing. He was drawing canal boats and different scenes he had seen over the following months that we had seen on the boat. This helped me to build his confidence in steering, which he enjoyed very much. He knew the safety rules on how boats should pass one another; to slow down if we were passing a moored boat, to slow down if he saw another boat coming in the opposite direction, and to steer the boat to the right position to pass correctly. Jonathan was thinking for himself and making decisions on how to proceed. This was wonderful progress and proved his capabilities.

I had ideas on how we could build on this new interest over time; this would help him in different ways and using his skills to progress. It would take time because of the cost of hiring the boat; although, at a reasonable cost, it still was a strain on my finances. Having learnt the basic rules on handling the boat, and realising Jonathan's interest in canal boats, I did not feel I had to hire the boat so often. Jonathan would always remember what he had learnt, and the time between going on the boat could be spaced out to help me save towards those costs without adding further worries and strain on my purse. I was always struggling to pay for any opportunities which I thought would be helpful to Jonathan. I knew I had to keep trying him with as many different activities as possible that might help me to understand his autism.

I felt I was doing all I could to give Jonathan a happy life with quality and opportunities to express himself. My fears for his future were never really out of my thoughts. He was making wonderful progress in many areas of his life but still not in his speech and verbal communication, or his willingness to try a variety of foods. I was understanding how his autism affected him in his daily life and structured our lives around his needs. What worried me constantly was his lack of ability to talk in more than two or three words. I knew he could read words, but not verbally talk in sentences. He was having daily mental stimuli to try and help, but speech did not improve.

His tastes in foods were still very bland and were of little variety. What he did eat had to be cooked and put on a plate in a certain way. This was an issue that I feared would be an ongoing problem for the foreseeable future. I knew that I had to try and change his rigid ideas about foods. I wanted to show him how to cook some simple foods that he liked, but I knew he wasn't at that stage in his development where he could understand. It was an issue which I intended to approach when the time was right.

Another idea I decided to try was to take him to a place to sit down and look at a menu to hopefully try something. Restaurants would be too expensive so I thought of going to a pub when it was quiet, to see if Jonathan would cope in an environment which was different from a fast-food outlet, and the choice of food would be healthier.

As Jonathan was approaching eighteen years old, he would be allowed in, and as we planned to be going at noon it was likely to be quiet.

I researched some suitable pubs and enquired about their menus. Having chosen one, I phoned the manager first to explain our situation and how Jonathan liked his food cooked and presented if he chose to eat (which at first, he may not) and would only have a glass of water.

I talked about the idea to Jonathan for a few weeks and waited for him to decide. The day came when he said, 'Pub for lunch.' I was so pleased he had been thinking about it and was willing to try. I quickly phoned the manager to remind him about Jonathan and checked that there would be food on the menu which he may like. As with everything about Jonathan's life I had to make sure things would go as smoothly as possible with what he was expecting to happen from what we had talked about.

Going into the pub eating area it was quiet and the table set out. There were one or two other people there but not sitting down to eat. I showed Jonathan where the toilet was and sat down to look at the menu. The waiter asked him what drink would he like. Jonathan answered, 'Water, please.' I felt that this experience may go well. I talked about the food on the menu and the meals he could try. Having spoken to the manager beforehand, he reassured me that Jonathan could have a meal prepared for him if he did not want anything from the menu. After going over the menu, knowing Jonathan would not choose the set meals, I asked him if would like an egg and some ham and peas, which he was happy about. When the meal was brought to us, Jonathan accepted it as the food was set out on his plate as I had requested.

All was going well and Jonathan enjoyed his meal; it was wonderful progress. As we were leaving the manager said goodbye to us and asked Jonathan if he liked his lunch. To my surprise, he replied, 'Yes, thank you.' On our way home we talked about the food and going again on another day. Jonathan said, 'Yes, again.' This was a big step in his development, not only his social skills but in his maturing. I knew we had a long way to go, but it was a step in the right direction for Jonathan being in an environment where he felt happy and safe, where people were friendly and pleasant to him, which he's very attuned to.

I knew I could build on this practice over time. We would not be able to do it every week due to the cost; something I was always having to take into consideration when introducing anything new to his routine.

As Jonathan felt happy about going out for lunch every few weeks to the same place, I knew it would be the right time for him to try a different place. Not wanting to stagnate and get stuck into a set routine I wanted him to experience eating lunch in a variety of places where he felt happy. I looked for other suitable pubs with eating areas and menus which Jonathan might like.

After making all the necessary enquiries before going to a new place for lunch, I felt that Jonathan was making very good progress. He was becoming confident about choosing meals from the menu, if he recognised a food item that he liked. The meals were not always a success as something might be cooked differently from what he was used to, but at least he was choosing for himself!

Having introduced the experience of going out for lunch, I had expanded his social skills, and he could cope a little more in the 'real world', which was my aim for him. It was progress that would help him to continue to develop those skills for the future.

I was building a life for Jonathan where he had a variety of activities he enjoyed doing, that were experiences helping his development and maturity; and being part of the 'real world' as much as possible within his capabilities.

I felt I knew I was doing my best for him and always had been over the years, without any help or support including from my daughter and her father. They had not been in touch to enquire how Jonathan was doing, which hurt me deeply because Jonathan had made so much progress, it was amazing to see! His communication skills were very limited, but I had hope that this would improve over time.

His ability to remember tasks, directions, road signs, and draw in detail were skills I wanted to develop as much as possible. Steering a canal boat and having to take appropriate steps of action when needed required coordination skills and being aware of what was ahead and around your boat. Jonathan was proving how capable he was. This motivated me to carry on and find other interests for him.

I felt that if he was able to make as much progress as he had, then his speech would improve.

I was doubting the way I had dealt with everything with not really understanding the full impact of autism. Maybe the ideas I had were not the right ones to help with his autism fully, but I knew they were helping Jonathan in so many other ways, and that was all I could focus on to keep me going.

At the heritage railway, the narrow-gauge was progressing slowly. The ground had been dug and levelled ready for the track to be put down. Jonathan continued to enjoy his 'work' there; he could see how it was coming together. He had worked hard at digging and clearing all the rubble. When track was put down the person overseeing the project knew that Jonathan liked using a special spanner to tighten the fish bolts which joined each piece of track together. He would make sure he did every one as he had been shown, then they would be checked. Jonathan was also working on an old miner's carriage which needed scraping and painting so that it could be used for passengers. It was a wonderful opportunity for Jonathan to be doing voluntary work on a hobby that he both was so interested in and felt a great sense of achievement doing. There was nowhere and nothing else available for an eighteen-year-old autistic young person to have such an opportunity.

The leader at the railway recognised Jonathan's capabilities and suggested that, as Jonathan was now eighteen, he could have a driver experience on a train on a day during the week when no passenger trains were running. I said that would be an amazing idea, but he would not like the steam train as it would be hot and dusty. The leader agreed that a diesel would suit Jonathan better.

He was confident that Jonathan would follow instruction from the driver whom he knew, and it was a reward for all the hard work that Jonathan had done. I would be able to go in the driver's cab too. When I talked to Jonathan about it, he was so happy and surprised. It overwhelmed me to see his reaction at wanting to do something I hadn't dared to think of or ask for, but for the railway to offer this experience for him made all the effort and belief in my son worthwhile!

Arrangements were made concerning the date and the time which Jonathan would be able to have his driver experience. The day finally came. Jonathan was excited and anxious, and so was I! The driver showed Jonathan which diesel train he would be driving. We got into the cab, and Jonathan sat at the controls.

The driver was known to us and was very friendly, and I explained I would find words which Jonathan understood if he got confused with any instructions. I intended to say very little as I wanted to see how much Jonathan understood of the instructions from the driver.

As he went through the controls, I could see how much Jonathan was concentrating and remembering that which he was being shown. The driver then asked Jonathan to turn on the engine and let the brake off slowly, remembering to sound the horn. Jonathan took the train out of the station slowly, listening all the time to the instructions. Then he was asked to go faster and use the controls which were required. To my absolute surprise he was driving the train on his own! The guard and the driver were amazed at Jonathan's skill at controlling the speed and changing gear when asked to. The driver instructing did not have to take the controls at all and he commented on how confident Jonathan was, remembering everything he was instructed to do. Braking was more difficult; bringing the train to a smooth standstill at the station was not easy. When we were approaching the station, Jonathan followed the necessary actions to slow down and brake smoothly to stop at the station platform correctly. I was overwhelmed at how well he did it; no help needed from the driver, who was surprised at Jonathan's ability.

When Jonathan had had several tries at driving that day, he became more confident and relaxed each time. When he finished his driving experience, Jonathan was very calm and felt a sense of achievement knowing he had managed to drive a train successfully. He had proven that if given the opportunity he could achieve so much. I was so happy for him and I knew Jonathan had 'grown up' that day. All the support and encouragement I had given Jonathan over the years was proving to have beneficial outcomes for him. He had driven a diesel train with very little assistance!

His wonderful memory and interest in trains could be developed and built on in the future to continue to make good use of these skills. I believe it was his autism that enabled him to have such ability, and I as his mother felt so proud of his achievements that it started to give me other ideas to keep moving forward. I always knew and had believed in my son, and I would keep trying the best I could to encourage and develop his skills further, with the hope that his verbal communication would improve.

My thoughts turned to my daughter Kelly and her father. I wanted so much to share Jonathan's wonderful experience with them, but I was afraid of their negative comments which would spoil the whole day. I decided not to contact them so Jonathan and I could enjoy the experience.

It gave Jonathan ideas to draw and write about; we talked about it for many weeks afterwards. The volunteers at the railway congratulated him on his driving, which helped his confidence. He felt part of a team doing a job and showed he was capable of driving a train too! All this was making it a worthwhile opportunity for Jonathan that I was extremely grateful to have found.

As Jonathan was now eighteen years old, I was informed by social services that he would be entitled to some funding. Not knowing about or understanding any of this, I had been struggling over the years by myself. I found out as he was now an adult, Jonathan could apply for funding for certain activities. This was good news, which could help me to find other suitable activities for Jonathan to do without me struggling so much financially.

When a social worker came to the house to explain all the details and gave me a list of places which held different activities for disabled adults, I asked about facilities for autistic adults, but the answer I got was, 'They deal with all kinds of disabilities.'

As this was all new to me. I was pleased that we would be able to meet others with similar disabilities, and hopefully build friendships, which had been a worry over the years. Although I had tried to find opportunities for Jonathan to socialise, making friends had been very difficult for him. Now, with social services giving us the chance to visit various groups. I thought that Jonathan's life would continue to improve.

Not knowing what to expect, I arranged for us to go and look at a group that did arts and crafts. It wasn't so much the activities which they offered, but I wanted Jonathan to have the opportunity to be with people his own age and to make friends.

Having arrived at the place where the arts and crafts group met, Jonathan and I opened the door into a large room with tables placed around and quite a number of people sitting and doing various tasks, with someone helping them. What struck Jonathan and I was the noise. I asked for the person in charge, who was in another room on the phone. She came out to meet us and was friendly towards Jonathan, who by this stage was getting stressed by the noise. We went into the room to talk about what the group did. I asked about the number of people in the room and the noise. She didn't seem concerned and informed me that they all got on well together. I knew that I could not leave Jonathan in the group.

I explained his autism and how he was not able to cope with noise and lots of people around him, and then I apologised and left! When we got outside, I felt shocked by what I had seen in the room. Those people were the same age as my son and yet they had different complex issues. They were sitting at tables not knowing what to do, as they only had a few members of staff to help them.

I calmed Jonathan down by reassuring him that we would not go back there again. I informed the social worker who did who did not show any concern or give any advice other than, 'Go and look at other groups.'

I couldn't face going to look at any other groups. My thoughts were stuck on what I had seen. I was angry and disgusted with the care those disabled people were getting! The hopes I had for Jonathan of making friends in an environment which suited him were dashed. All sorts of questions were going through my mind. Was this the level of care I had to accept for my son? I couldn't understand that if those people had been in a school over the years, why was their behaviour so challenging as a young adult?

I had been working so hard with Jonathan to help him improve with so many of his difficult issues. Seeing those people in that room made me realise just how much progress Jonathan had made. To put him in a group like that would have had detrimental effects on his development.

After a few weeks I decided to go and look at another group which would welcome members, who were outside on a small animal farm. I thought this would be more suitable and enable Jonathan to have some contact with animals such as chickens, rabbits, sheep, small goats and horses. Members would learn to look after the animals. There would only be a small number of members on any one day. When Jonathan and I were looking around, the person who was in charge was talking to Jonathan about feeding the animals; he would need to wear wellington boots and old clothes as he may get dirty. She showed him inside a purpose-built barn where there were washrooms, a dining area for their lunch, an activity room to draw, and rest. It all seemed just the place which would give Jonathan the opportunity to learn different skills.

Having talked with him about going there for one day in the week he seemed quite happy, as he still went to the railway to do his voluntary work. I felt that this could help Jonathan. Working with animals and not many people around him, with staff who seemed interested in helping him, would encourage his social skills.

I informed social services that Jonathan wanted to go to the farm for one day a week. They agreed funding, and the date was agreed on for him to start. I was extremely anxious about letting him go but I knew the time was right for him to try. I had explained all about his autism and his reactions to certain situations, including his likes and dislikes about food. They reassured me that the cook would be aware when preparing his lunch.

The day came for Jonathan to go to the farm. He had a bag with his trousers and boots to change into, and he knew what he was having for his lunch. When I felt he had settled in it was time for me to leave and I returned at 3 p.m.

Those few hours from 10 a.m. seemed to go on forever!

I was worrying about him. I couldn't settle to do anything. When the time came for me to go and pick him up, I felt relieved and happy when I saw how relaxed he was. The manager said he had done very well feeding the animals and had eaten his lunch of sausage and beans.

When we got home, I asked him what had he been doing and what he had for lunch. I felt we had found another opportunity that could help Jonathan. It involved animals which we didn't keep at home, nor would we ever be able to. Over the following months he was doing a variety of tasks very well at the farm and was not afraid of being close to animals. When I turned up earlier than expected to pick him up, I could see just how he was coping around animals, which was wonderful to see. Jonathan was also making friends with the few members that he knew. Only having small groups meant social skills and confidence could improve. I was grateful that we had found such a calming environment for Jonathan, and I did not have to worry about the cost.

I felt Jonathan's life was becoming varied, and giving him opportunities to develop in confidence, communication and independence skills!

As time passed, I began to notice that Jonathan wasn't quite as interested in going to the farm and didn't seem happy when I picked him up in the afternoon. When I mentioned this to the manager, she gave me several reasons and tried to dismiss my concerns. I knew my son was not happy, and I had to find out why. One day I decided to go earlier to pick up Jonathan to see how he was coping. When I arrived at the farm, there was no one about, so I went into the barn. As I got through the door, the noise was deafening. There was screaming and shouting from a member who was upset about something, and two staff members trying to calm that person down. They looked shocked at seeing me and carried on dealing with the issue. I quickly looked round to see where Jonathan was and went into the activity room. There I saw quite a large group of people sitting, standing, walking around, shouting, getting stressed; no staff with them. I was angry and worried because I still couldn't find Jonathan. I went outside and started calling him and I saw a shed door open where they kept boots and coats for changing.

I went in and saw Jonathan sitting in a corner by himself looking frightened and upset. I calmed him as much as I could and tried to find out what had happened. He couldn't tell me but I worked out that the noise from the member inside was too much for Jonathan to cope with. No-one saw him leave the barn and go into the shed. I helped Jonathan change his shoes and got his coat to leave. As we were walking out of the ground another staff member came running to us trying to explain the situation. I asked why there were so many people in the group, when they had said it would always be small groups. I informed them that I would be reporting what I had seen to social services. My son would not be going back!

When I got home and calmed Jonathan down, I tried to talk about what had happened. He said, 'Too noisy.' I was upset and angry with myself at not finding out sooner. My instincts told me something was wrong, as Jonathan wasn't happy going, but he couldn't tell me why.

I phoned social services and they explained that there was not enough staff at the farm that day, as it was so popular lots of people chose that day to attend. My concerns about safety and suitability were dismissed. I informed them that Jonathan would not be going back there.

I was again shocked, angry, and could not understand why such a wonderful opportunity (as it had started as) could turn so quickly into a situation where large numbers of disabled adults with different needs, were expected to cope in an environment with not enough staff to supervise, or deal with complex challenging behaviour of some of the members, who clearly were unable to cope with being at the farm.

I began questioning myself and my expectations, not only for my son, but for the other people I had seen.

Before social services had come into our lives, I was trying to give Jonathan the best quality of life I was able, and as many opportunities to help him develop. Having experienced what society had to offer our disabled adults, I was disillusioned and worried about his future. I decided I did not want to try any more groups. Jonathan needed to settle in himself. We went to the railway, where he could get on with his 'work' and was learning too.

Going to the farm did help him at the beginning to be involved with animals, and showed me how he was able to carry out all the different tasks that needed to be done, so it was an experience, if only for a short while, which was invaluable. I was upset that Jonathan could have done so much more there, but he couldn't cope with the large groups, and there wasn't enough for all the group to do, therefore, a great deal of time was spent sitting around with nothing constructive being done.

When social services came out to discuss the problems we had experienced at the farm, I explained that my understanding at the start was that they would only have a small group to enable members the opportunity to care for the animals and to socialise with other members. Jonathan was happy for the first few months, and I had seen how he enjoyed interacting with members whom he knew, and coped with feeding and cleaning out the goat stables and other animals. As I had seen him doing all his tasks over time, I felt reassured he would go on to develop his skills. Then he began to be less happy about going. I hadn't noticed how many new members had joined, because they came at different times. When I tried to ask Jonathan about his day. He would go very quiet and not want to talk. I also asked him about his lunch, but again, I had the same response. That is why I decided to go earlier one day to find out what was happening.

The social worker explained that the farm manager was hoping to have more staff but was not in a financial position to do so, as they were only just starting the centre. I was surprised that social services were willing to pay for people to go there, and yet they were aware of the lack of staff with the number of members, all with different disabilities. The social worker informed me that the cook was finding it difficult to get Jonathan to eat anything. I questioned why I had not been informed about this. I was made to feel it was my fault, that I had been 'expecting too much'!

I decided it was no longer the right place for Jonathan, and told the social worker I would carry on finding opportunities for my son, as I could not accept what they had to offer.

We carried on visiting different places to go out for lunch every few weeks. Progress was being made with his choice of foods, being able to cope with going to a new place and feeling confident, and feeling grown up in himself too!

My thoughts would return to those groups and people I had seen. I could see the ones who had some autistic traits which Jonathan had when he was younger, but he had overcome and managed to deal with them. Yet these were adults of the same age or older than Jonathan, who had very challenging behaviour. I wondered about the schools they went to, and it made me realise that the decision I had made to take Jonathan out of the system, as hard as it had been and continued to be, I knew was the right one.

I accepted that his social skills were affected, but he couldn't socialise anyway with his sensory issues. They had to be worked on before he could move forward in his development.

Now, he was getting to the stage of being able to cope in the 'real world' and in environments that suited him and his needs.

I was always looking for new opportunities for Jonathan to experience, and having seen what was on offer for disabled adults, it made me more determined to find activities which suited him and *his* needs; not just expecting him to fit into groups that he couldn't cope with.

One day I saw in the newspaper an advert for adult beginners who were interested in archery. Coaching on a one-to-one basis was available, with equipment supplied at the club.

I read the advert several times and I thought about how Jonathan might like to try it. Again, I was thinking about his hand-eye coordination skills. I spoke to a coach about Jonathan's autism and he explained that the club encouraged all disabilities, were trained to show people, and would decide if new applicants were suitable from a safety point of view, which I fully accepted and appreciated.

When I talked to Jonathan about going to try archery, he was very happy about the idea.

When the day came to go to the club, I was very nervous inside and wondered if I was expecting too much of Jonathan. I just wanted to give him opportunities.

The people at the club were friendly, and the coach who was going to work with Jonathan introduced himself, showed us around the club, and looked at some of the different archery equipment. The coach knew from our telephone conversation how to explain to and physically show Jonathan everything that he needed to do. The safety rules were practised over and over again. I could see how Jonathan was listening and remembering what he was being told by the coach. When the time came for Jonathan to try to use a bow and arrow, I watched closely how he went through the safety procedures with the coach. When the coach asked him to let go of the bow and try to look at the circle on the target board, Jonathan thought for a short while and released the bow. It was a wonderful first try, and the coach was surprised at how Jonathan had grasped what he needed to do. After several tries, I could see this was a skill that Jonathan seemed to like, and it showed how his coordination had improved over the years.

I was amazed and happy for him, because this was something where verbal communication problems would not cause him too much difficulty. It was concentration, hand, arm, and eye coordination that was important. Despite having never been in an archery club before, or understanding how difficult archery is, the coach said Jonathan had the ability to do well at archery.

Over the weeks Jonathan looked forward to going to the club and was making good progress. The coach informed me that they could apply for a grant from the Disabled Sports Association for Jonathan to buy his own equipment, which would continue to help his progress with the sport. I was so pleased and grateful for the help, as I could not afford to buy any equipment and I was struggling to pay for the course, which I felt would benefit Jonathan to have the experience, as with any new activity he had the opportunity to try.

When the grant came through for his equipment, the coach advised us on what to purchase. Jonathan felt confident and happy to have his own equipment, just like the other people at the club.

The coach was pleased that he could help Jonathan obtain a grant and commented on how getting used to his own bow would make a positive difference.

Jonathan was enjoying going to archery each week, and I felt he was progressing well. I was amazed how he would focus upon the target and was determined to get the bullseye! When I watched the other experienced archers there, I saw that Jonathan had learnt very fast, and had surprised both the other people and the coaches. I was encouraged to learn the basics of archery, and safety issues, as anyone who went into the club needed to do.

After trying myself to use a bow, I realised how difficult it was and appreciated Jonathan had managed the skill.

With his voluntary work at the heritage railway (which he enjoyed very much) and learning a different sport, I felt that he was doing the things that suited his needs, and was making progress too.

Continuing to expand his social skills by going to different venues for lunch every few weeks and exploring other heritage railways at weekends, I felt I was doing my very best to give him a meaningful life with quality that still took into consideration his autism.

My thoughts turned to the activities that social services had to offer and it started to make me feel very depressed and despondent about my son's future. I had been working so hard over the years to help him manage his autism and to overcome the many difficult situations, with a great deal of time and patience and love! I wanted my son to have a life doing things he *could* do and enjoyed. The shock of reality and lack of opportunities for disabled adults filled me with despair. All I could do was keep trying to encourage Jonathan in every way possible. This was my aim and intention as a mother.

I had not heard from social services for at least six months when I received a letter informing me of another day care centre which Jonathan might like to try.

After getting all the information from a visiting social worker on this centre, which offered sports, cooking, arts and crafts, and life skills, it sounded very interesting. Not rejecting the offer straight away I said I would talk with Jonathan about it, and we would go and have a look to see if he was happy to do so. I was assured groups were small and one-to-one sessions were available in different activities. I decided to read through all the paperwork before making an appointment to go and see it. I did not want to upset Jonathan and set him back in his progress, which I feared would happen again.

Thoughts were going through my mind about what sort of centre it would be like, and if it was offering everything it said on paper.

I felt guilty that if I didn't let Jonathan try it, I could be holding him back. He needed some independence from me! But I knew it had to be the right place for *him*.

After a lot of thought and talking with Jonathan about going to have a look at the new centre, he seemed willing to go and stay for a little time. After making the arrangements about a date and time and giving as much information as possible about Jonathan's autism, they were confident that he would like it. The day arrived when Jonathan and I went to the Skills Centre, as it was called. The staff were friendly and showed us around the building. It had a big kitchen where students learnt to cook and eat with other students. There was an art room with lots of equipment, and a room to look at books and to relax. There was a garden which students looked after. It all appeared very nice, and there weren't many students in any of the groups. Jonathan was made to feel very welcome; this helped both of us. After looking around the centre, I had lots of questions to ask. One question I asked was whether Jonathan could bring his own food to learn to cook at lunchtime due to his issues with eating. The manager said that was a good idea and a staff member would supervise him cooking. He could also go to the local gym on a one-to-one session if he wanted to.

There seemed to be a variety of opportunities, but I was still hesitant about Jonathan going. I needed more time to think it over, and maybe take Jonathan along for another visit to see his reaction. The manager understood my concerns, having heard about the experience at the previous day care centre.

As the Skills Centre was out of our area, I had to work out the travelling costs and time it would take to get there and back if Jonathan decided to go. Although the day costs were funded, travelling costs were not. As with any activity which would be of benefit to Jonathan, I had to find a way of adjusting my financial commitments to pay for it.

After making another visit to the Skills Centre, Jonathan seemed willing to give it a try. A start date was arranged for one day a week. The day arrived for Jonathan to go. He had his food packed which he wanted for his lunch, and he would be helped by a staff member to prepare. Having explained everything again at the Skills Centre about how he liked his food, I asked if he could be supervised to do it himself as much as possible. I felt reassured that Jonathan would settle and enjoy his day. I couldn't relax after leaving him there, and I was so anxious about how he was coping. I phoned the centre after lunch time to ask how he got on, they informed me that Jonathan had enjoyed his lunch and would be doing some art in the afternoon. I could not settle until it was time to make my way to pick him up. When I got there, he seemed quiet, but I expected that it was because everything was 'different' for him. On our way home I asked him about the things he had done and asked him if he wanted to go back again. He said yes, which helped me to feel better that I had made the right decision to let him try the centre.

I wasn't sure what I had expected from the Skills Centre, other than Jonathan having the opportunity to socialise and have a little independence from me, even if it was just one day a week.

He enjoyed going to the heritage railway to 'work', and I felt that now Jonathan was getting a variety of meaningful opportunities and making wonderful progress.

We visited different heritage railways on Saturdays and Sundays, which enabled Jonathan to use his skills at map reading, finding his directions, and understanding of road numbers, signs and timetables to plan journeys to somewhere he liked and knew what to expect when he got there. Heritage railways operated in the same way.

Continuing to help him with his social skills and trying new foods; he enjoyed going out to lunch every few weeks, which I felt was encouraging him to overcome his eating issues. I accepted it would be an ongoing exercise, and I had hopes of the Skills Centre helping him develop his cooking skills. They had the facilities and worked with small groups, which would help build friendships and social skills while cooking and eating together. I felt this was as important as doing other activities.

After a number of sessions at the Skills Centre the manager suggested to me that Jonathan would benefit by going for another day, if I could get the funding from social services. As I wasn't sure if it was possible regarding funding, I asked about the things he would be doing if he went for another day. The manager said he could go to the local gym on a one-to-one basis and he could continue to develop his cooking skills. I thought both suggestions would benefit Jonathan if he wanted to go for another day, and if funding was available.

I approached social services about funding before I asked Jonathan about wanting to go for another day. Also, I had to work out the travelling costs. After a few weeks, social services informed me that they would fund another day.

Having spoken to Jonathan to find out his reaction and explaining what he would be doing, he seemed pleased about the idea. I let the Skills Centre know of the funding and agreed another day on which Jonathan would go.

I was optimistic that the centre was going to prove beneficial for him, and they understood my aims for his progress, which reassured me about Jonathan going. I was feeling settled in myself that his life was becoming varied and structured to suit Jonathan's needs.

As time passed, I was hoping that Jonathan would progress in confidence by going to the Skills Centre, but each week there would be a problem, either with not having sufficient staff to supervise the cooking of his lunch, with the food items Jonathan chose to take with him to prepare, or problems at the gym, and various other reasons why Jonathan's routine had not been followed. I began feeling disappointed again at myself expecting too much. I put every effort into helping Jonathan settle in and he was looking forward to doing the activities which he had been promised in his care plan. As I could not afford to travel back and forth each day he went to the Skills Centre, I would stay in the area and go to a library and to take the opportunity to find out any information about autism, and ways to help my son.

I was prepared to do whatever I had to, to give Jonathan the experiences which may benefit him, only to be faced each week with Jonathan being upset at not having the lunch he wanted, or not doing the activities he was expecting to do. The lack of understanding from the staff at the Skills Centre of how important routine is to an autistic person made me very angry and frustrated!

I felt guilty about making the wrong decision again about what I had thought, and hoped, would be the place to help Jonathan with his skills. I had been working on this with him for years without any support, only to find that it could not offer what they said at the start of the introduction. All it came down to was numbers of people attending to obtain funding. There was no real concern or aims for those disabled people attending other than giving them 'somewhere to go for a few hours',

After having a meeting with the manager and social worker and expressing my disappointment with the centre and the lack of training for people with autism, I decided Jonathan would not continue to go there. It was wasting his time when he could be doing more constructive things. I had tried my best to work along with the centre, only to have my son's development set back again, which I was not prepared to let carry on! After a year of attending the centre, Jonathan had not learnt anything of any benefit. I had to make up for all the time he had wasted.

Jonathan was happy in himself when I explained that he would not be going back, and he would go to the heritage railway and do his work, where he was learning constructive skills, and I would continue with his eating issues by going out to different venues for lunch. I also intended to try taking him to a gym to encourage his physical skills, and to find out what the problems were, which the staff at the Skills Centre couldn't deal with.

Although I was angry and upset that it hadn't worked out at the Skills Centre, it made me realise that very little was expected of disabled people, and opportunities for them to progress were limited. I had tried over my son's life to search for new things for him to explore, and continued to encourage and support him to develop in as many ways as possible, only to be faced with reality, where there were no expectations or encouragement for him to progress.

Jonathan was approaching nineteen years old and had not made the progress I had hoped for, despite spending the time at the Skills Centre. I felt absolutely frustrated, angry, upset and most of all guilty because I had let him waste so much precious time there thinking that maybe things would improve, and doubting myself about what I was expecting from them. I knew my son could achieve more if he was given the opportunity and support, but I was made to feel that I was an overprotective and pushy parent, which brought all the fears I had about my son's future to the surface again. Only this time I started to get very depressed and frightened about the future.

I had been trying over the years to understand my son's autism and effects on his daily life, to find ways to deal with his complex issues, and hoping to meet others who could help me with encouraging Jonathan to progress; people who would have the understanding, respect, and motivation which autistic people are attuned to and respond to. I felt total despair about how society and professionals expected so little of them. Again, I was alone, and I had to reject that which social services were willing to fund just so that I had somewhere to send my son two days a week—without any positive outcomes. But I was not looking to send my son anywhere to get him out of the way; I wanted quality care and support with his progress as the outcome! I asked myself over and over again, 'Is that so wrong?'

I had really struggled over the years, financially, emotionally and physically, doing the very best I could for my son. When he became an adult, my hopes were raised of help from social services offering some funding, which I could use to find ways to help Jonathan further. Instead, it was disappointment and despair.

After explaining how I felt to social services and informing them that I did not want any more funding for places unsuitable for my son's needs and I would continue to support him myself, they accepted my decision and said that they would keep in touch if I changed my mind.

It took several weeks for Jonathan to settle down, and he seemed relieved at not having to go back to the Skills Centre again. I was very low in myself, not really knowing which way to go anymore.

All my son had was me, who loved and cared for him, and was willing to try anything and go anywhere, no matter what the cost, to help my son progress, and have some quality of life that took into consideration his needs.

How could I expect society, social services, or any day care centre to be really interested in my son when his own father and sibling, whom we hadn't seen for many years, didn't care about his progress or even want to help him? I began to doubt my capability as a mother and what I was trying to achieve, against all the obstacles I had faced, and still battling to overcome. I felt alone and scared.

The diagnosis of my son's autism had consumed my life, trying to understand how it affected him. I realised that the professionals or society did not know very much about it, nor even as much as I did, of the effects it had upon the person, close family, or the devastating consequences. No one seemed to care!

Having reached a very low point I knew I had to accept that it was only my enthusiasm, motivation, love and devotion that could help Jonathan, however difficult and upsetting it was. I had to find the strength and courage to carry on, for my son.

I started going over in my mind all the things he couldn't do as an adult. Lack of communication skills, sensory issues, not being able to socialise in groups or make friends, his appetite problems (which was a growing concern), his need for routine; his issues seemed to affect his whole life, and were making daily living difficult with no hope for the future. I felt a complete failure, not knowing which way to go. I found it hard to focus on anything positive, but I knew I had to keep trying, for my son's sake. This deep depression made me accept that even with all the devotion I had tried to give Jonathan over the years, he would always need help and support, and that realisation scared me.

All he had was me, who was trying to understand autism as best I could, and not to let it get in the way of giving Jonathan the best quality of life possible. It hurt me very deeply to find out that society did not have the same aspirations for people with autism as I had, and I found it extremely difficult to accept.

Again, I would realise how little my son's sister and father expected of him to progress, so how could I expect society to be any different?

Feeling angry and disillusioned with people, I felt that my belief in my son's capabilities would prove over time that progress was possible, and by giving him the opportunities, he could achieve.

I continued to work on his reading, writing and communication skills. His self-care skills were improving, which would be ongoing throughout his life. I knew I had to try and get some help with his eating issues, but I was not sure where to go. I was worried about his emotional and mental health, as he couldn't verbally express himself to describe his feelings when he became frustrated and upset about something. I had to try to find out what the problem was, which wasn't easy! And at times, asking him questions would make him more agitated. I would feel very upset at not being able to help him. As an adult his emotional wellbeing was worrying me, but not knowing anyone else to talk to; it was up to me to find a way of coping with an autistic adult.

My thoughts turned to his physical health; his lack of vitamins from not eating enough nutritious foods.

As much as I encouraged him with different tastes and going out to try foods from a menu, his lack of appetite was not improving, and I knew I had to do something. I went to a health food shop to find out about the cost of vitamins. The assistant at the shop was very helpful and gave me some leaflets about items which could be useful. I was starting to understand that Jonathan may be lacking in certain vitamins; this could be contributing to his emotional frustration. This was an issue that I felt was connected to his autism and needed attention.

After reading the information from the health food shop, I decided to try a wholewheat loaf with no additives. It was something I felt would be a start, encouraging Jonathan to eat a food that he liked toasted or as a sandwich, and it had no additives. It cost more than a supermarket loaf of bread, but it seemed a good way of introducing a healthier food. I could only afford to buy one a week. Although Jonathan could taste the difference from his usual bread, he did eat it after a while, which I was so pleased about. We went to the shop each week to buy the loaf of bread and I was getting more information about foods that may help him which did not have additives. The whole concept of Jonathan's eating issues and lack of vitamins, or reactions to certain additives in the foods he did eat, was making me think about the idea of it somehow being part of his autism, or in causing him further problems. I wanted to find out as much as I could about it. I went to the local library to find books which might help me.

On a usual visit to buy a wholemeal loaf of bread from the health food shop, a customer who was also buying bread started saying how her health had improved over time since she had changed her eating habits and began to eat foods without additives. I was very interested in what she was saying. She gave me the name and telephone number of an herbalist consultant who had been a great help to her, and who was also an iridologist. He did have a clinic locally and had a very good reputation.

I decided to phone the consultant to get more information, to ask if the treatment could help Jonathan, and to find out the costs.

I wanted to learn about anything I thought would help my son.

After a lengthy conversation with the herbalist, I decided to make an appointment for Jonathan and me to visit him. The appointment date I made gave me a few weeks to talk about it to Jonathan, and for me to work out my finances to pay for it. I had to juggle household bills, or miss paying certain ones, as I had always had to do, to give my son every opportunity I could which might help him.

As I had felt let down by his doctor, who had shown no consideration or understanding about my concerns for Jonathan's health over the years, as a result I could not see the point in causing Jonathan or myself further stress by making any appointments, only to be offered drugs to 'calm' him down, which I *refused* to accept as a solution.

The day arrived when we were going to see the herbalist. I did not know what to expect, or what information I would be given because it was all new to me. When we got to the room Jonathan became very anxious, worried that it was going to be like visiting the doctor, which he did not like.

The herbalist was very pleasant, quietly spoken, and made us feel very welcome. His room was bright, soft colours, and no smell of anything that reminded Jonathan of a clinic. There were pictures of eyes around the room, and a camera and laptop on the desk. He explained that by looking closely at the eyes he could see if there were any health issues that herbal medicine may be able to help with. After finding out about Jonathan's medical history, he asked him if he could take a photograph of his eyes and then show him them on the laptop to explain his findings. The herbalist involved Jonathan as much as possible in the discussions to try and understand his emotional health and to see how he reacted when stressed in new situations.

After taking a photograph of his eyes and enlarging the photos on a computer. He explained that Jonathan had allergies to certain foods, which would cause him to have digestive problems and affect his appetite.

Jonathan's system was almost always in a stressed state, which would make him irritable as he couldn't explain how he felt.

The herbalist needed to take into account Jonathan's emotional and mental state, so that he could give the medicine which suited Jonathan's needs. I was amazed and fascinated by what I had learnt, and it all made sense to me.

I was so relieved to have found help for Jonathan with his eating issues, and his mental and emotional health, which his doctor had not even talked about. I felt if Jonathan could become calmer, it would have beneficial effects on his whole wellbeing, and maybe he would move forward with his appetite. My hopes of showing him how to cook healthy meals, which he liked, was now a possibility in time.

Having finished the long consultation, the herbalist said the bottles of medicine would be posted in a few days. Jonathan would need to take the number of drops as stated each day for a few weeks. Any changes would be gradual, and I was to make any notes which might help at the next appointment.

When the medicines arrived, I had to encourage Jonathan to take them, which was difficult for the first week, but then he began to feel less stressed each time he took the drops on a spoon with a little water. I tried to get him to count out loud the numbers, which after a time he liked doing. I wasn't expecting any changes to happen, but I felt hopeful that Jonathan might start to feel better.

As time passed, I could definitely notice that he was becoming calmer. There weren't any significant changes to his appetite, but he was starting to eat a little more of the foods he chose. I tried not to draw attention to it and always praised and encouraged him to finish his meal, which wasn't always successful. We talked about healthy foods and looked at books about foods our bodies needed, and about cooking different healthy meals. I felt I had to continue with the topic as it was an issue that affected him in many ways, and we both needed to understand how certain foods affected him, and to find out about foods which might suit him better with nutritional benefits.

I was so relieved to have found someone who could explain what Jonathan's problems were. Although the consultant did not give any definite hopes that Jonathan's eating habits would greatly improve, he did reassure me that helping his mental and emotional wellbeing may encourage him to enjoy his food without him becoming stressed by worrying about how it could make him feel. I knew myself over the years it was a complex issue with Jonathan, and it concerned me greatly that I had no one to discuss it with. His doctor showed no interest in my worries over Jonathan's eating problems; the lack of care for and understanding of autistic people is why I had lost confidence in the health service.

The herbalist-consultant was interested in my son's wellbeing, and he felt confident that herbal medicine could help Jonathan over time, which gave me hope as a mother. I had found another way to help improve my son's quality of life. I was determined to overcome obstacles that at times seemed insurmountable.

As a mother of an autistic adult, I began to feel I had explored as much information and had enough experience to understand how it affected my son's life, and finally, had found help to hopefully encourage him to eat foods which were healthy and would not have ill effects. I was also hoping to work towards helping him prepare and cook meals he liked, which would develop his independence skills as well as his appetite. I accepted it would take time, as with everything over Jonathan's life, but it was another goal to aim towards, with positive outcomes.

We were continuing to work on all the activities that we had been doing; reading, writing, numbers, clocks and planning journeys to heritage railways or other places of interest, and self-care skills.

We were now at the stage where Jonathan was learning about healthy eating. My aims of showing him how to cook meals he liked himself, with supervision, would be a huge step in his development and independent skills, which I had hoped for but never thought a possibility until I found the help and understanding from the herbalist consultant.

Although I accepted my son would always need support, I wanted him to be able to do as much as he possibly could for himself. As a mother, I felt so strongly about him not being completely dependent on someone for his food, or self-care. His dignity and respect as a person were very important. Having experienced the centres, day care activities that social services had to offer, it worried me greatly that disabled people's feelings were not considered.

Jonathan continued to enjoy going to archery and the heritage railway working on the narrow-gauge project, which was progressing in its development. The idea of Jonathan doing another driver experience at another railway seemed like a good way of continuing his progress and enjoyment of his skills, and ability to adapt to different people and trains.

I decided to begin enquires with the aim of Jonathan having the opportunity to experience driving other trains with supervision. As they were expensive activities, they would be goals to work towards for Jonathan. I also wanted to find out about gymnasiums which we could go to and work on his physical health and coordination. After searching for a suitable gym and giving them information about what I was trying to help Jonathan with, I found a gym that wanted to help and suggested that Jonathan and I have an introduction there. An instructor would spend time with us showing us how to use the equipment. I thought it was a helpful suggestion. After arranging a date and time, I talked to Jonathan, who was very anxious about going because he remembered his experience of going to a gym with a member of staff at the Skills Centre, and it wasn't a happy time. I wanted Jonathan to have a positive experience of going to a gym.

The instructor showed us around and how to use the different exercise machines. Jonathan was encouraged to try the various machines for himself.

My concerns about him going into the changing rooms by himself were alleviated by the instructor who explained that they had a changing room for disabled people and that he could use that. I started to feel hopeful with this new activity and all the new skills Jonathan could learn. I realised that the staff at the Skills Centre did not put any effort in to help my son enjoy going to a gym, and I would need to encourage him. It gave me another opportunity to learn new skills *with* Jonathan, whilst helping his physical health and coordination skills. I felt that I was doing my best trying to take in all of the learning issues my son had due to his autism, while continuing to explore new activities to help his progress whilst giving him the best quality of life possible that I could give him.

It still worried me very much about his lack of communication skills. Jonathan was approaching twenty years old but still had problems with speech, language and communication. He was making progress in many ways with issues affecting his daily life, but not in his speech, which would start the worries and fears I had for his future.

As a mother, I wanted to help and do everything I could to give my son every opportunity that would make it possible for him to progress.

Somehow, I still felt I was failing him, but with hope, love and devotion I had to keep trying!

Chapter Five
Twenty to Twenty-Five Years Old

We started going to the gym and working on Jonathan's coordination, and physical health. With him being more active, I was hoping his appetite would improve over time. I felt that the herbal medicine was helping Jonathan to feel calmer and that he would continue to make progress there.

As we were able to go to the gym quite early in the morning, this meant that there were fewer people present. This helped him to settle and to enjoy his exercise. As time passed, Jonathan looked forward to going and was making progress with each exercise. He learnt very quickly how to use the walking machine and adjust the speed which he felt happy with, and with the rowing machine he knew what strength setting he wanted.

When we went into the squash court to do bat and ball skills, I would speed up the ball to try and encourage his reaction skills. It took time but I began to notice progress. We weren't playing by any rules because he didn't understand the rules of a game; we just enjoyed running about to bat the ball. This was my purpose for the exercise. It did help to alleviate my depressive mood a little.

He was gaining confidence by going into the changing room himself while I waited outside. At first it would take him quite some time to get changed into his gym clothes, but as his confidence improved, he was taking less time and would come out feeling quite independent. This was a big step forward in his development.

It was these moments which made me feel so happy for him. This helped me to realise that I was giving him every opportunity that I could to continue with his progress.

It was difficult but I had to accept that my son, who was now twenty years old, would not be able to live the life of someone his age who did not have autism.

He would always need support. As his mother, I had to help improve his independence and communication skills to give him a happy, quality life, with opportunities for him to achieve.

I felt very alone, not having anyone to talk with about my worries and concerns for Jonathan's future. I accepted that it was I who had made the decision to take my son out of the system and to try and do my best to understand his autism. I could not accept knowing what the health or education authority had to offer. After going through many difficult years that affected me mentally, physically and financially, to see the progress Jonathan had made proved to me that he *was* capable of achieving if he was given opportunities and support. I had to learn every single day of his life how autism affected him and how to try and help him to cope with his life. When he became an adult and social services informed me of groups and centres, they funded which he could go to, I had the hope of Jonathan being able to make friends in an environment doing activities he enjoyed while being supported, only to be faced with the reality that society had so little expectation of people with autism. I began to doubt myself as a parent and questioned myself over and over, 'What am I trying to achieve with Jonathan? What makes me think that I can understand autism?' Then I had to remind myself that I had lived autism for all of Jonathan's life! I knew how it affected him and what needed to be worked upon every day.

I was not prepared to accept poor quality care for my son, and I would continue to do the best I could to help him progress!

I continued to work on the main basic skills: sensory, coordination, reading and writing, self-care and appetite. We learnt about healthy foods, with the aim of Jonathan being able to cook meals with support. The herbal medicine had positive effects and enabled Jonathan to cope with daily life and problems he had.

I felt I was acknowledging every single issue that Jonathan needed help and support with. Many times, it has been heartbreaking to have to admit to myself that my son cannot live a 'normal' life, so we have had to cultivate a life which suits him, however abnormal that may seem to the outside world, and that is what I have tried to do.

I became more frightened of Jonathan's future when he hit adulthood due to my experiences of how society had so little understanding of autism, with few opportunities to help them progress and achieve. I knew I had to keep finding new activities and encouraging Jonathan by myself as I always have.

Neither my daughter or my children's father made an effort or wanted to help and neither would expect Jonathan to have made the progress which he had. I was hoping that we could have worked together to give him the support he needed for his future. I felt as though the moment I made the decision to try and help Jonathan and not accept that which was on offer at the time of his diagnosis, I had been left to get on with it. My daughter and her father could not understand the love and devotion of a mother to help her child, and society did not care either. I knew very little about autism, and the professionals were not able to advise me on how to help my son, as they did not understand autism either. I was on my own but I was willing to try, and that was all I could do as a mother.

The heritage railway project that Jonathan was helping with was almost finished. I had made enquiries about doing a driver experience at other railways. After explaining the situation of Jonathan's autism and his ability to remember what he is told or shown to do, some heritage railways were reluctant to give him that chance. They could not understand autism. I tried several railways until I found one that did understand and was willing to give Jonathan the opportunity, which I was so pleased about. I wanted to make people aware of the amazing ability my son had in the hope of raising awareness for others in the future and breaking down the fear people had about autism.

I managed to arrange a date at a heritage railway that Jonathan and I had visited before, so he was familiar with the surroundings, and what trains were there. When the day arrived for Jonathan to do his driver experience, he was excited but stressed because he didn't know the people there. I knew it would really test him mentally, physically and emotionally, but I felt he was ready to try.

That experience would show me the progress Jonathan had made and how he could cope with people he didn't know instructing him. When the driver and guard introduced themselves to us, I felt that Jonathan was at ease with them. I stayed in the driver's cab with Jonathan and observed how he coped with the instructions given to him. I had explained in detail before that day to the driver and guard how to use words that Jonathan could understand and remember. I was so pleased that they were helpful and caring to make sure Jonathan had understood their instructions. After the day had finished, we were both very tired and extremely happy at how well Jonathan had done. The driving instructor and guard praised Jonathan for his efforts and for listening to every instruction they gave and his careful control of the train.

Although it had been a very expensive day, it was worthwhile! So much had come from the experience; Jonathan felt confident and had a sense of achievement, which made me realise how capable my son was! It was another experience I could expand on. I was always looking for ways and opportunities to help him to progress.

I was planning his next driver experience and finding out about other forms of transport which did the same. I came across a museum for tramways. Again, not knowing if they offered driver experience days, or if they would consider my request, I phoned to get details. To my surprise, they would allow Jonathan to have the opportunity to drive a tram, because he had driven diesel trains. After explaining his autism and how to show him what to do and what words to use when instructing him, I felt confident that Jonathan would cope with this new form of transport. The Tramway Museum accepted my request for Jonathan to drive a tram! I felt as though I had broken through another barrier of helping others to try and understand autism, or at least not to be afraid of people with it, and accept that people have the ability to learn if they are shown understanding and kind consideration.

These new experiences were testing Jonathan and proving to me, he was capable of so much more!

I felt he had a quality of life which was taking into account all of his issues on a daily basis but was still giving him opportunities to work towards proving his ability to learn and enjoy experiencing activities which encouraged his skills. He was losing interest in archery as time went by. The coach wanted him to enter competitions and travel to other clubs to compete. Sadly, I had to explain that Jonathan did not understand competition or rules of a game. When he had gained the skill of a sport, that was enough for him! Winning or losing didn't mean anything to him. As that activity came to an end, I began looking for new ones because I did not want him to stagnate in his development.

As his coordination skills improved, he needed to try different activities to help him to continue to progress.

The next new activity that I thought would help his coordination was golf. Again, not knowing anything about it, I made enquires and found a driving range located near where we lived. I introduced the idea to Jonathan and we decided to go and have a look. He really enjoyed having a go at hitting the golf balls. I spoke to an instructor who advised that a one-to-one lesson would help Jonathan learn the safety rules and how to use a golf club. After asking about the cost, I decided to arrange for him to have some lessons to see if he would like it. When the day arrived for Jonathan to have a lesson (with a very understanding instructor) I was amazed at how quickly Jonathan was learning the basic techniques. The lessons were at a reasonable cost which enabled Jonathan to have one each week. I wanted him to be shown the correct way by an instructor and knew that he would remember every detail. The lessons at the driving range had helped Jonathan when on the nine-hole golf course and he enjoyed it very much. I observed and tried to take in as much as I could. I knew I would not be able to afford the ongoing lessons for too long, and I would be supporting Jonathan when going round the course.

After a few weeks the instructor suggested Jonathan try going around the course with me. He was confident that Jonathan understood the safety rules and needed to practise on the course. The instructor commented on Jonathan's coordinated hand and eye skills, which was important when playing golf. That comment made me realise that persevering and working on his coordination skills over the years had helped him to progress. I felt that having another new activity to include in Jonathan's routine would have positive outcomes for his physical and mental health. Being outside in the fresh air in a peaceful environment was wonderful for us both. We enjoyed going several times a week to the driving range if the weather was too wet to go on the golf course. I could see the concentration Jonathan showed when trying to hit the ball at a target, and his sense of achievement if he managed to get it right.

I felt so happy for him; it was wonderful to see the skills he was progressing with. It would also make me feel sad that his father and sister had missed out and not had the expectation or hope that Jonathan was capable of so much, and still had more to develop! As his mother I always believed in his ability to learn, although his speech and communication skills were still of real concern to me and I knew that I must keep trying to encourage and help to find new ways to continue to help him develop.

His stress was becoming less, which I felt was because of the herbal medicine. Jonathan began taking an interest in me showing and encouraging him how to prepare and cook simple meals he liked. He would write down all the meals which he chose for one week in his notebook and complete the shopping list for the items. I encouraged him to draw pictures of the foods he liked and how to prepare each item, building up a folder of pictures of healthy foods. When supporting him using the cooker, I would go over the danger issues within the kitchen and how to cook foods slowly, always reminding him of safety. He was very particular as to how his food looked and was presented on a plate. After supervising the cooking and making sure it was properly cooked, I encouraged him to put the food on his plate as he wanted it, knowing that he would then eat it. Learning to prepare and cook simple meals was going to be a long process, but I felt confident. As with everything with Jonathan, it all had to be done at his pace, and each day if he managed to accomplish a new task like peeling potatoes, cutting carrots or cooking an omelette, it was a step forward in his development and independent skills, which had always been my aim and intention.

I believed my son could achieve more as long as he was given the opportunity!

Jonathan had a constructive, varied life, and I felt that he was happy. I was trying my best to keep focusing on helping him to progress as much as possible. But, deep down inside of me, I would worry myself into a state of despair and depression, when the realisation came into my mind that Jonathan would have no one to care for him if anything happened to me. His own father and sibling had rejected him, and we didn't have any close friends or relatives to help.

My thoughts turned to social services and the fear of what kind of life they could offer him. This frightened me. I just wanted to help Jonathan be as independent as much as he could, but the possible future filled me with dread. I felt that I had failed my son, and I couldn't understand what more I could do than that which I already had been doing.

Not having heard from social services for a year, a letter arrived saying Jonathan was due for an assessment for funding. It stated a date and time when a social worker was due to visit us. I didn't feel positive or hopeful about anything they might have to offer. Past experience had proven it to be a waste of time for both Jonathan and me.

I wasn't sure whether to cancel the appointment; Jonathan was happy and contented and making progress in his life! After giving it a great deal of thought, I decided to go ahead with the meeting to find out what they had to offer. I wanted to give Jonathan every opportunity, and I did not want to let him down by not accepting an offer that could be of help to him. I talked to Jonathan about someone coming to see us, but that he would not be going anywhere he had gone to before like the Skills Centre, which still held bad memories for him.

The social worker was pleasant, hadn't met us before, but was aware of all the problems Jonathan had experienced at the previous day care centres. After listening to find out all the different activities Jonathan was doing, she realised that there was nothing more social services *could* offer regarding activities.

However, after giving me information about changes in the system for disabled adults, I could have support workers for a certain number of hours each week, who could take Jonathan to any of his activities and support him in enjoying his interests. This was information about changes I wasn't aware of and I had lots of questions about safety, capability of the support workers, funding, and general suitability.

It sounded like a very good way of helping disabled adults gain more independence but I was concerned about how much experience they had, particularly with autism. The social worker assured me that all support workers were police-checked and given training before being given any clients to support. I was interested in finding out more because I could understand how it may help Jonathan in his independence, social and confidence skills, if he had the right person supporting him.

It gave me hope of my son being able to meet other people who were there to help him. I tried not to get too optimistic, not because of the thought of letting another person care for him (although, that did worry me) but because I was unsure what experience these people would have with autism. I had devoted twenty years of living with autism and was still learning!

The social worker gave me the phone numbers of agencies they used and advised me to contact them to arrange for suitable workers to visit us before making the decision to involve them in Jonathan's life.

After contacting several agencies recommended by social services, and getting as much information as I could,

I decided that I would try having support workers as long as they were the right person to care for my son.

Our Experience of Support Workers

After meeting a few support workers who the agency thought would be suitable and Jonathan seemed to like, it was for me to decide which activities they were going to support Jonathan in doing. I explained to each one about the different things Jonathan did. I decided to introduce them to the heritage railway so they could understand his interest in trains and get involved with him. My hope was for a support worker to take him one morning a week, and I the other. The person chosen was shown around the railway, and the work shed where the tools were, plus the kitchen facilities. I suggested they came along for a few visits until I felt comfortable with leaving Jonathan with them and that he felt happy about it. I explained all the safety issues about the railway and the work Jonathan was doing. I expected the support worker to want to get involved. I encouraged the person to work along with Jonathan doing whatever task he was working on. Instead, the support worker would just stand watching him, not interacting with him at all! I asked the person if they had a problem with being at the railway, to be told that they didn't like it and knew nothing about trains. It shocked me that they had no understanding of what was expected of them when supporting someone in the community.

I reported this to the manager of the agency and asked them to only send people who had an interest in their role as a support worker. This was a new experience for Jonathan and I. I thought that maybe we could get someone who was interested in their job and was understanding towards my son.

After meeting several support workers that the agency said would be suitable, I showed each one what Jonathan liked to do at the heritage railway. To my disappointment none of them were interested in supporting him with the activity, and I did not feel that my son would be safe left in their care.

I expressed my concerns to the manager and declined to have any of the support workers they had recommended to accompany Jonathan at the railway. I also asked about what training they were given as none of them knew anything about autism. The answer I got was that they had all had 'in-house training'!

I found it very difficult to accept that social services were paying people to do an extremely important job, and yet the support workers who were sent to us had very little interest in what they *should* have been doing, or how to support an adult with autism. As much as I had tried to explain what Jonathan liked doing and the help he needed for his own safety, it became obvious quite soon that these support workers were not adequately trained.

After more lengthy meetings with social services about my concerns and disillusionment on the capability of the support workers, I was astounded at the attitude and accusation that I might be expecting too much of them! All I was asking for was support workers who I felt I could leave my son with, where he would be safe and happy.

That comment made me doubt myself. I felt maybe I hadn't given the support workers guidance about what they should be doing when supporting my son. I started blaming myself.

I had devoted my life to helping Jonathan, and had cultivated a life doing different activities that he liked and was making progress in. Having the opportunity to have support workers help gave me a little hope of Jonathan gaining social and independent skills with other people who were motivated as I had always been. I tried to justify the support workers' lack of interest as a response to being at a railway. As the project had completed and there were no tasks to do that suited Jonathan, we would spend more time at the gym or golf.

As time passed, I thought about the experience of the support workers I had met and decided to contact other agencies to find out what they could offer, because the idea of Jonathan being supported was a beneficial one, if only he could get the right person.

Now his railway project had finished, maybe we could find someone to support him at the gym or golf.

I had done all the foundation work, and Jonathan was happy and confident at those activities. I decided I must try again with the hope of finding the right person.

After contacting several agencies, they all said their workers were trained and their job would be to support the client in whatever activity the client chose. It was not up to the support worker to decide. I got more information from the agencies and possible workers that may be suitable.

Interviews were arranged for Jonathan and me to meet them. I explained it would take several meetings to help Jonathan feel at ease with anyone who was suitable, and funding would have to be confirmed by social services before any support could begin. There were two different people I thought may be able to support Jonathan; one to go to the gym, and the other at golf. I explained to each of them how I would introduce them to the activity until Jonathan felt comfortable with them, and I was happy about them caring for Jonathan.

After funding was agreed and the dates arranged to start work, I tried to feel optimistic and help them to interact with Jonathan. Although his communication skills were limited, he could still show his feelings of stress or contentment, and I needed the support workers to understand as much as possible about his autism, for them to be able to cope whilst supporting and keeping him safe.

The date was agreed that each support worker would join us at the gym or golf. I talked to Jonathan about what would happen when the person joined him for the activity, and I would stay with him and show the support worker what they had to do. I was trying to be optimistic for Jonathan's sake. I felt that he was trying his best to cooperate.

The day arrived when the support worker was going to join Jonathan and me at the gym. When we got there, early in the morning, comments were made as to why it had to be done at that time. I explained that was what suited Jonathan.

After showing the support worker how the machines worked, which ones Jonathan liked to use, and their safety issues, I accepted that it would take several visits before the support worker could show me that they were motivated in helping and encouraging Jonathan. After a few weeks of me observing how the support worker was getting on, I decided to start leaving them alone together, though I would wait outside. At first, it was ten to fifteen minutes, then I increased the time until I felt that Jonathan was confident and happy being alone with the support worker.

When the time had been built up to an hour, I decided to ask the support worker to take Jonathan to the gym by themselves. I felt that I had shown the person what was expected, and Jonathan was happy having that person with him (which pleased me) because he was feeling more independent. It was an extremely difficult and worrying time for me, to let him go, but I knew it was his independence I was aiming towards.

The first few months went by without too many problems, and I began to feel optimistic. Then the support worker started letting Jonathan down by not turning up on time, which was very important to Jonathan. I would often get phone calls to say that their car wasn't working, or other reasons for not turning up. Jonathan did not know from week to week if they would turn up. I was prepared to take him if he was to be let down. After quite a number of times of being let down I informed the agency that I did not want that worker anymore. The agency told me that the support worker didn't like going to the gym early in the morning. Jonathan could use the walking machine by himself, and he did not interact or talk with the support worker.

I was angry and upset at such a comment from a support worker who had no proper training, other than that which he had been given on how to help my son, and that he couldn't engage in conversation because of Jonathan's communication difficulties.

I was becoming exasperated with the role of support workers. I began to feel frightened of the future for Jonathan. He was trying his best to cooperate with them and enjoy his activities, but he could sense their lack of interest.

The frustration was starting to affect my mental health and again it was making me feel depressed. I was doubting my own capability as a mother.

I knew I could not accept the lack of interest or training of what social services called support workers.

My thoughts turned to my expectations of the care I wanted for my son, but I started to realise that might be impossible to find.

The idea of having to accept poor care for my son was something I would never be able to do. I kept hoping things would change!

I knew I had to give the support worker who I had chosen to help Jonathan at golf the opportunity to try, which I did, and went through all the safety issues and how to encourage Jonathan and interact with him. I was prepared to guide that worker for as long as was needed before I felt confident to leave Jonathan in their care. The support worker had shown an interest in the sport (which I was optimistic about) and Jonathan got along quite well with the person. After a number of visits with us at the driving range and nine-hole course I felt that it was time to let them go by themselves.

The support worker used to turn up on time to take Jonathan to golf, and they both seemed to get along with each other, which raised my hopes of asking the support worker to help Jonathan in other activities. I decided to wait and see how things went on. One particular occasion when Jonathan was expecting to go to golf with his support worker, the weather was cold and damp, but Jonathan wanted to go and had the waterproof clothing. The worker didn't seem keen on going and tried to suggest that they do something else. I explained that the driving range was under cover, and if the weather permitted later, the nine-hole golf course should be open.

I had a nagging feeling that something was not right with the attitude of the support worker. After reluctantly agreeing to go, I decided I would go later to see if Jonathan was alright. As it was raining, I expected them to be on the driving range. When I got there, I could not see them, and I asked at the reception desk (where the people knew Jonathan and I) where they were.

I was told that they had not been in yet. I was angry and worried because I did not know where my son was! I tried phoning the mobile phone of the support worker, but there was no answer. I phoned the manager of the agency to inform them, who agreed that it was against their policy rules and they would register my official complaint. My concern was for the safety of Jonathan, and I was going to inform the police, which I did straight away. The police came out to the golf club to get more information. I began panicking with fear and anger and blaming myself for letting it happen knowing these support workers had absolutely no idea or training or common sense when they were supposed to be caring for vulnerable people.

I was advised to go home in case they had gone back there as the weather was still wet and cold. When the time came that they were due back, the support worker's car pulled up outside. Through sheer anger I ran out and opened the door to Jonathan and got him out. I raised my voice at the worker to find out where they had been, saying that I had informed the police and the agency. The answer I got back was, 'It was too cold for golf, so we went to town to look at the shops.' I slammed the door and went inside to make sure Jonathan was alright. I asked him where he had been, to which he said, 'The shops.' I tried to get more information later and I accepted they had gone to certain shops, although Jonathan was unhappy about going. I reassured him that there would be no more support workers and that I would take him to golf and the gym.

My official complaint was given to the police and the agency and to social services to take the necessary action, if any was to be taken! I had several meetings with social services and made sure that my complaint was registered at the highest level, and that the lack of training of support workers was an area that needed urgent attention involving the county council, who would also be made aware of my complaint.

I had lost complete trust in the system and I decided I would continue to care for my son myself.

Feeling very angry and despondent with the whole experience of support workers, I became very depressed and wondering, how much more my mental wellbeing could take. I felt completely alone and feared for my son's safety.

The future consumed my thoughts constantly. I blamed myself for thinking that everyone should care for vulnerable people in the way I did. The realisation of how society cared left me feeling scared for my son's future. I knew the concerns I had raised regarding the training of support workers would not be listened to or acted upon. I was just a lone mother who had gone against the system, to try to do the best for her son herself, without any help or support from anyone.

After coming to the decision to have no more support workers, I knew I had to try and cope with my fears to continue helping Jonathan as I had always done, on my own. I focused upon all the issues as I had been doing over the years; sensory, coordination, reading, writing, self-care skills and working to support Jonathan in preparing and cooking meals he liked.

He enjoyed going to the gym and golf, which was having beneficial effects on his physical and mental health. Always looking for new activities to expand his skills, as with his train driving experiences, I was giving Jonathan a varied, structured life, which took into account his needs.

As another year had almost gone by and Jonathan was making progress in his development and maturity except for his speech and communication skills. This was a concern and a great worry to me because I just didn't know what else I could do to help him. Approaching twenty-one years old, I was hoping that more progress would have been made, and I couldn't understand why it hadn't. He was happy in himself, which I felt was very important, and his confidence in willing to try new ideas was improving; I related this to the beneficial effects of herbal medicine he took daily as part of his routine. It was having a noticeable effect enabling him to cope with new challenges. The herbal medicine was working on his wellbeing; his mind and personality. How he saw the world! I knew if I kept encouraging his development that his communication skills would improve, and I would find other ways of helping him.

Sometimes an idea or thought came into my mind that felt right to try with Jonathan. On one particular occasion, I had turned on the radio in the kitchen whilst Jonathan was preparing his lunch. A song was playing which I liked and I began to sing along to it. For a few moments, I felt a sense of being happy, and Jonathan was enjoying preparing his food. That was the moment I got the idea of singing. If I could find songs he liked and encouraged him to sing along, it might help his speech!

Each day while Jonathan was preparing his lunch, I turned the radio on and talked about the songs and encouraged him to try and sing along with me. He didn't show much interest at the beginning, and the songs playing weren't always ones he liked. This gave me another idea of getting a CD player and looking for songs he may like. It was something I felt strongly that we could expand upon, and I felt sure it would encourage his speech.

After buying a CD player, I started to look in charity shops for CDs because I couldn't afford to buy new ones; especially not knowing how many I might need before I found one Jonathan liked. We went each week to a charity shop to look for CDs; sometimes I found one or two which I thought that he may like, and other times there wasn't anything suitable. As it was a new idea, his interest in music had to be encouraged because he had no experience of any artists or groups that he liked. Choosing a CD was difficult, so I listened to what I thought he may like. As with anything I introduced to Jonathan, I knew that it would take time, which I accepted, and kept trying. When one day we did our usual visit to the charity shop, I found a CD with songs from the sixties. There was a variety of songs for him to choose from.

When we got home, I put the CD in the player while helping Jonathan prepare his lunch and observed his reaction to the music. I didn't sing along to any because I wanted to see if he liked any of the songs. Having got almost to the end of the CD, a track by Nat King Cole, 'Wonderful World' was playing. The words were easy to listen to, and Jonathan stopped what he was doing and went over to the CD player to turn the volume up. I was amazed at his reaction when he said, 'Again.'

He wanted to listen to it again. I was so happy and surprised at the choice of song that he chose and we played it a few times. I knew then that something wonderful had been achieved in his development, and it could be built on. He was then able to connect going to the charity shops and looking for a CD with other songs he may like to listen to. If he did come across a particular song he liked, I wrote it down in a notebook, because I wanted to get an idea of what type of music was resonating with him, like Nat King Cole, Johnny Mathis, Elvis Presley.

Jonathan was enjoying the experience of listening to music but did not want to sing. I had the idea that if he had the lyrics to the songs, I could encourage him to sing along.

I was getting very excited and hopeful with the whole idea. Jonathan had an interest which helped him feel calm and happy; this had not been possible in the previous years due to his auditory and other sensory issues. Also, his stress levels were now being helped with his herbal medicine. I felt that by working on those areas over the years, and continuing to do so, Jonathan had now reached a stage where his development could be progressed further, in the hope that his communication skills improve.

To help this new interest I needed a computer to find lyrics, as it would take time to go to the library. Not being able to afford a new one, I decided to apply to a charity which helped disabled people with grants for equipment or aids.

Having searched for possible ones to which to apply to, I was very surprised when my application was accepted and

I was given a small grant for a used computer, which was wonderful. I could go forward with helping Jonathan to develop his interest in music, which was having beneficial outcomes.

Having a computer enabled me to find and write out the lyrics to the songs which Jonathan liked. I put them in a folder and I would read through the lyrics line by line encouraging Jonathan to say each word of a song, turning it into a part of his reading routine. When he listened to the CD, I would encourage him to sing along and follow the lyrics. It wasn't easy for him to follow the words and sing along to start with. Although he could read the words, he had to think about using his voice to sing, which he found difficult.

I realised why his communication skills were causing him difficulties, and it was connected to his auditory issues. His sensitive hearing was becoming more manageable for him over the years, because of the continued work on that issue; but listening to his own voice was a completely new experience for him. Having found that he had an interest in music, something that I had not thought of during the difficult years when his behaviour and stress levels were challenging, the information the clinic had given me where I took him to as a child all made sense to me regarding his hearing and how it affected speech.

Jonathan found singing and hearing his voice a strange experience. He had no idea of how to sing high or low, but he tried to sing. This was showing me had the ability to learn, and it was helping me to understand more about how his autism affected him. Music was another way of helping him in his development and gave me hope.

To expand his interest in music, I bought a used amplifier and microphone. The idea I had was to encourage Jonathan to sing by himself, to me, at home. I chose one afternoon each week, because then I hoped it would be accepted as part of his routine activities. The equipment would be set up together with his lyrics and CDs for him to choose his songs. It took quite a lot of encouragement to get him to try one or two songs. That is all he would attempt at the beginning. Again, hearing his own voice through a microphone was strange for him, and he would turn it off. I felt confident over time that he would enjoy singing and using the microphone. Until he felt happy about it, I would encourage him to sing along with the CD following the lyrics. As he got used to the weekly afternoon of music, he would often turn on the microphone for a short time. This showed me that he was feeling more relaxed with the activity. Also, he would extend the number of songs he sang. The connection between following the lyrics and listening to the song on CD was being made; that was progress, and I knew that he had got over another hurdle in his development.

The next stage in expanding his skills was to encourage him to write out the lyrics to songs he had chosen. He enjoyed doing that and numbered them in order for his folder. I showed him how to list them by number so that he could find the one he wanted more easily.

Jonathan was starting to spend more time looking for the lyrics to different songs, then writing them out to put in his folder. We continued going to charity shops to look for CDs.

He progressed from visiting the same one to understanding that other shops may have ones which he may like. Over time we had got quite a variety of CDs; Jonathan was enjoying listening to different songs, choosing ones which he liked, then writing out the lyrics for them.

Although he had a varied, structured life which was cultivated to suit his needs, the introduction to music and singing was having positive outcomes I hadn't expected, and I felt happy for Jonathan to have got to the stage where he could enjoy music, just as anyone else does who isn't autistic. It made me feel that he was doing something 'normal', which most people took for granted, but life for Jonathan, living with autism, nothing could be taken for granted. Everything had to be introduced and learnt at his pace.

Progress was being made in his development as I continued to work on his coordination, self-care skills, reading, writing, cooking skills, healthy eating, sensory and other auditory issues. Finding a new interest that was helping his confidence and speech was also having a calming effect on him. I knew it could be expanded to help Jonathan in many ways.

Each week we both looked forward to our afternoon of music; it was relaxing for me, because I hadn't had the opportunity for many years to listen to music. Jonathan was gradually singing along to his CDs and following the lyrics. I could hear when he was having difficulties singing a word and help him to pronounce it when he read over the lyrics again. Music was having a noticeable positive effect on his mood, and I felt the same uplifting feeling which Jonathan did. It made me realise how important music and singing is for our mental health.

I was always looking for new activities for Jonathan to experience which would help in his development. His social skills were limited as he could not cope in large group settings, and all of the activities he had been doing over the years were ones which he could do on his own with me supporting him. Making friends was not easy for Jonathan due to his autism and lack of communication skills. It was a real worry for me that he could not socialise; there weren't suitable opportunities for adults with autism.

As Jonathan was becoming more confident with singing, I had an idea of expanding the activity by going into the community and hiring a hall. It would encourage him to sing in a different environment. My hope and intention, was, to see if other adults with similar disabilities wanted to join us.

I knew Jonathan was enjoying music and singing; maybe we could meet other people to form a small social group. The idea seemed a way forward, to form our own group. I knew it would take time to develop a group where Jonathan and others could socialise in a safe and happy environment, that took into account their needs. Even though I had not done anything like that before, I felt confident about trying to do it.

After searching for rooms to hire, I found a church hall which charged very reasonable rates. When I put the idea to Jonathan, he wasn't happy about it, because he could not understand why we would take our equipment out of the house to go somewhere different. We went to look at the church hall several times, and I talked to Jonathan about where his music things could be set up for him to sing. The idea was not accepted by him! I began to doubt if it could work and if I was being too optimistic about forming a small group to help Jonathan to socialise.

I decided to take all the things on another visit to the hall and set it up, to see if it would help Jonathan to understand that he *could* sing in another place. I played a CD he liked and tried to make the environment relaxed. I encouraged him to sing along.

After some time, when he realised that it was just us two in the room and he had walked around to find out where the toilet was and saw there was a small kitchen for him to get a drink of water, he started to calm down. I had to wait for him to feel comfortable and safe in the environment before he would take any interest in his music. We hired the hall on the same afternoon and time he would normally sing at home. It was something I felt I had to try, without knowing if or how long it would take him to accept it.

The first few weeks were difficult for him to get used to going to the hall. The sounds of the music and hearing his voice through the microphone was different in the bigger room. He didn't like turning the volume up!

Over the weeks I realised that there were a number of problems regarding sounds, and how the bigger room was making the music sound different to Jonathan. I tried changing the position of the equipment in the hope of finding the best position for Jonathan to feel comfortable with it.

At times the whole idea seemed hopeless and I wondered if I should accept it was not going to work out because of the sounds and their effects on people with autism.

Although Jonathan's hearing had become a little less sensitive over the years, his new experience of singing using a microphone and hearing his own voice was raising other issues regarding sounds and effects.

As I was feeling less optimistic about going to the church hall, I suggested to Jonathan that we could sing at home. To my surprise, he said, 'No, go to the hall!' I knew after many weeks of trying he had accepted singing at the hall, and I felt he really wanted to go.

That afternoon was enjoyable for us both. Jonathan seemed relaxed and adjusted the volume to which that he felt comfortable. He used the microphone more confidently. He had made another step forward in his development, and it gave me hope that we may be able to form our own group to meet others with similar disabilities, where they could socialise in a safe and happy environment!

Jonathan had got to the stage where I felt the time was right to try and see if other people with similar disabilities wanted to join us. I had some leaflets printed with details of time, day, and a short description of what we did and suggested that if anyone was interested to bring along their own CDs to enjoy. I knew it was important, learning from Jonathan, that people with autism had their own things and did not like anyone touching their possessions.

Having put some leaflets in the local library, churches, and a few shops, I didn't know if any interest would be shown, but as with everything I tried to help Jonathan with, it all took time.

After a few weeks went by with no contact from anyone, I began to have doubts about the whole idea, but still felt that it was the right way to go for Jonathan. I was determined to carry on, because we were both enjoying our 'music time' at the hall.

After quite a number of weeks had passed and no one had shown an interest in joining us, we arrived one week at the hall for our usual music time, and outside were four people waiting by the door! I observed that two of them had learning issues and the other two must be support workers. I asked who they were looking for and they said, 'The group that does music!'

I was so pleased that they wanted to join our small group, where they could socialise and enjoy listening to music. I asked if any of them had brought their own CDs. They hadn't but would listen to Jonathan's music (which they seemed to enjoy). I was encouraging Jonathan to sing because I knew that he was a little anxious with strangers in the hall when he was used to just the two of us. I tried to involve the two people who wanted to join the music group. Not knowing them, and not wanting to make them feel nervous, I had to rely on their support workers to help them to join in. When it was time to finish, I wasn't really sure if they wanted to come back again, but the support workers said that their clients definitely enjoyed themselves and would come back next week. I felt happy for them and pleased that they wanted to come back!

It was going to take time for Jonathan (and anyone else we met) to get used to each other. It was my intention to take everything slowly, so that everyone could settle and feel happy and safe in the environment, enjoying music, which would help their social skills. Having the experience over the years of understanding Jonathan's autism, I knew what kind of environment they could cope in, and be themselves in. Ensuring everyone felt happy and part of the group, singing their favourite songs, would have positive outcomes.

Keeping the group small in number was the most important point. People might have had different tastes in music, plus a calm atmosphere had to be maintained, with no loud sounds which would cause stress and anxiety. I knew the vision I had for the group, which could help Jonathan and others to socialise in a safe environment where they could enjoy an activity that could have so many beneficial effects.

By meeting others who enjoyed being with us and wanted to come back proved to me that my vision and hope of going forward in developing a group was the right way to go. Not only for Jonathan, but for others too!

Over the following weeks, the two new members were settling in, and Jonathan was accepting that they were there. I kept encouraging a little social interaction between them each week as I got to know the members more. If they brought their own CDs, I would suggest that each member take turns to listen to their chosen song while the others listened.

Slowly, I was starting to structure each session with small steps, taking turns with CDs then encouraging each member to interact with Jonathan by taking their CD to him to put into the player, and saying which track number they wanted.

I was finding new ways each week to help them make eye contact with each other, which is a difficult issue for people with autism. Jonathan had to get used to trying to understand others and what they wanted. I wanted to encourage teamwork as much as possible, and as the weeks went by, I could see progress in their confidence and social skills, which made me realise that this was the right way to go.

Jonathan was gaining confidence and wanted to help the others in the group by operating the CD player and by taking the CD back to the person to whom it belonged to, when the song had finished. I purchased a notebook to encourage Jonathan to write down the name of each member in turn, and the song they wanted to sing or listen to!

This was encouraging structure and cooperation between the members, which they liked and felt happy with. Autistic people need order and organisation for them to feel secure and safe.

As time passed the small group was proving to me that it was helping the members to socialise confidently, and to be themselves. Jonathan would write in the book each week the songs the members wanted, and it was accepted that he would put the CD in the player and return it to the owner. The group was evolving in a wonderful way which I knew could continue to expand; not in numbers, but in opportunities!

I was becoming more aware that the support workers who accompanied the members were quite happy to let me organise each music session, and to encourage members to take part in whatever way they were able. I was so focused on making sure members enjoyed themselves and interacted with each other, I didn't really mind that the support workers were not getting involved, because I was understanding the new members and their needs more.

I accepted that anyone who did join our group would probably need to be with a support worker. I needed to help them understand what I was trying to achieve for my son and others too. I felt relieved that the support workers were not caring for my son, thinking about the experience with them that we had had. I was developing the group to suit Jonathan's needs and the needs of others who had joined us. The support workers seemed to just bring the person to us, taking little interest in getting involved, and letting me guide and encourage members as best I could. Any attempt to involve them to interact was refused, and comments made, that their member was doing alright without them. I felt that the support workers did not understand how I was trying to develop the group.

They just saw it as somewhere to go for a couple of hours each week, and left me to organise the session while they sat and did nothing! I did not want to raise any issues that may result in the members not coming, who were enjoying being part of the group and gaining in confidence.

Thinking of ways to continue to expand the skills of the members in our group, I had an idea of trying to use musical instruments, and to find out if they liked any particular one. Giving thought to sounds and noises that people with autism and learning disabilities might find distressing, as I had learnt over the years from Jonathan's issues, I decided to get a tambourine and two maracas. As I couldn't afford anything too expensive, I started to look in charity shops for suitable instruments. Having managed to find a tambourine, maracas, and a xylophone, I felt sure that Jonathan and the other members of the group would enjoy having that opportunity to make their own sounds. It would also help me to learn about which instruments they liked. When I introduced the instruments and encouraged them to try and make their own sounds, Jonathan or the other members did not show any interest; they just wanted to sing or listen to their music!

I understood and accepted that anything different to which they usually did would be difficult to begin with for them to want to try. I left the instruments on a table so that the members could use them if they chose to, in their own time, however long that took.

Over the weeks, I would play an instrument whilst encouraging the members to sing along and to try to develop their interaction skills. Being a small group, it enabled me to get to know the others more, and to understand their issues.

The support workers were not helping the members and would just sit and watch whilst I encouraged them to use an instrument and join in. I knew that it would take time for Jonathan and the other members to enjoy interacting and using musical instruments, because they hadn't had the opportunity before.

In a short time, Jonathan had moved forward from singing at home to going to another place where others joined him. It was wonderful progress to see him and others becoming more confident and starting to work as a team. This was proving to me that I had to carry on with my hope and vision of developing a group where people living with autism or learning disabilities could go and socialise in a safe and happy environment.

As I got to know the members and understand their issues, I was finding ways to encourage their confidence. Autistic people find it very difficult to make eye contact with others, so when they arrived at the group, I would say to Jonathan, 'Let's go say hello to…' and we would greet each person. When going home, I would say to Jonathan, 'Let's go and say bye to…' This was helping them all to be sociable to each other, and to feel part of a team. I felt that this was very important for the group to develop and to respect one another, even with their learning issues, I knew from caring for Jonathan, that they had the intelligence and ability to learn if given the opportunity and respect from others.

Each week I could see progress from Jonathan and the others in confidence, cooperation, and communication. The musical instruments were being used more and I was encouraging them to dance and move to the music a little.

I had observed that coordination was a problem and would try swaying to the music or clapping or playing the tambourine. I was hoping the support workers would get involved, but they showed little interest. I had to accept this and stayed focused on that which I was trying to achieve at each music session.

I continued to look for other instruments in charity shops, and for CDs which I thought would be of interest. I did find a guitar at a reasonable cost, and to my surprise Jonathan seemed to like it straight away. He couldn't play it, but liked to hold it and pretend to play. When I showed him how to use his fingers on the strings, he didn't like the feel of it, and just wanted to hold the guitar.

Although Jonathan's sensory issues caused him to dislike the feel of the guitar strings, he pretended to play it. Using his imagination was showing me that he was progressing in his development.

People with autism find it difficult to use their imagination. To them they learn through what they see and remember. When Jonathan was a child, he could not understand imaginary play as children without autism do. The members who had been coming to the group each week had got into a routine of how they chose their songs, and to take turns to listen to the others. Jonathan wrote in the notebook the names of the songs, and whose turn it was. This structure was helping them to work together; being a small group, it enabled me to encourage each one. I was very pleased that Jonathan and the others were getting to know each other more too. The support workers, who changed every few weeks or so, did not show any motivation towards the people they brought to the group. This did frustrate me but I was glad that I could focus on developing the group to benefit all the members.

As time passed, I had other enquiries from parents and day care centres for people to come and see if they liked it. I explained that I could only enable one or two at any time because I had to consider the members who were already part of the group and how they may react to strangers coming in. I was understanding more how I believed that the group needed to develop, to take into consideration the members' needs. It was not my intention to have a large group because I knew it would not have the positive outcomes I was seeking. As I was doing this voluntarily, it had to be something I could manage! I had no expectation of any help from the support workers. After making arrangements for new members to join the group and explaining to the others that someone else would be visiting us, it prepared them. This was so important to people with autism and learning disabilities. It gave me the experience of meeting others with similar issues to Jonathan, and to see how their support workers interacted with those they were supposed to be supporting.

There were one or two new members who I felt could settle into the group. I gave them time to see if they were happy in the environment or not. I had a list of others I could contact if a place was available, as I kept the number to six people.

As the Christmas season approached, I began to think about having a party for the group, taking into consideration the likes, dislikes and issues each member had, as I had got to know them better over the months. I felt that it might be an experience for them to have a seasonal celebration which suited them, and not what society would expect them to like as being 'normal'.

After giving it a great deal of thought and asking the support workers if it was possible to bring the members, they agreed that it would be a good idea.

Then I talked about it to the group to get their reaction. As I expected and understood the members didn't show any interest, because it wasn't Christmas yet—as it was November, it did not have any meaning for them.

I knew the hall I had hired was going to put up decorations at the start of December, which I hoped would help them to accept and feel part of the season.

Jonathan did not like talking about Christmas before December, as I had had experience over the years about how autism affects the way they see things.

I started planning how to structure it a little more around our normal music session. The food each person liked, and what small gift I could get for the members suited to their likes. I thought about introducing one or two games to help them interact with one another, and to promote eye contact as much as possible. I wanted to make it a happy occasion which took into consideration their needs.

Jonathan had not been able to cope with social situations, and over the years had become isolated. This was the reason I wanted to develop the group to give him, and others, the opportunity to enjoy themselves in a calm and happy environment, which I felt was being cultivated within the group.

I had been paying for the hall myself and purchasing the instruments and had to work out the costs for the party. I felt it was something I wanted to do for Jonathan and the other members. Although I was doing the group voluntarily, and had made this known to parents and support workers, there was no offer of any contribution towards the cost.

As December was upon us and the hall was decorated for Christmas, I talked each week about Christmas songs and party games, food, and presents. Having got CDs from charity shops with Christmas songs, I introduced one or two to the group to find out the ones which they liked. I accepted they wanted to listen to their usual songs, but I gradually got them to listen to Christmas ones too. We talked about foods each person liked. It helped me to plan the party around them. I tried to keep up the motivation each week, preparing them that on the day of the party, we would be doing different things too!

I managed to get a small gift for each member as a surprise. I made sure to have the foods which suited each member and hoped that they would be eaten! There was a lot of preparation for the occasion, but I was happy and excited to be able to do something special for the group.

Jonathan was coping with the talk of the party and the expectation of what would be happening. This was progress for him as he had not been able to socialise or build friendships before, because he could not find anywhere which suited him. Now, after forming the group, the members were ready to have their own party. I wanted everything to be right for the members, as I felt this was a huge step forward for both Jonathan and the others. It also started me thinking more of the future of the group, and how I wanted to develop it with more instruments and equipment that might help with issues autistic people have difficulties with. I had a vision for my group but it was clear to me that I couldn't do it without funding in the new year, I was determined to make enquiries to find if it was possible to get any funding for a group which needed to remain small, to give autistic people the opportunity to socialise and to develop in confidence, communication and teamwork skills. I wanted the group to have a name, as everyone is an individual and different. The name I felt described that, and the one I would go forward with is:

Uniquely Me & U

The party went very well and I was observing all the time the reactions of the members as I encouraged them to sing along to a few Christmas songs. I introduced a very short and simple party game and encouraged each person to join in. I understood the difficulties each one had trying to follow the game. I kept the instructions simple and short so each person could feel part of the game even if they didn't understand what to do. It didn't matter, because I knew from caring for my son that he couldn't follow the rules to a game, so my intention was for them to be happy and for me to learn how I could help them! The food was enjoyed and I observed how each member chose their particular favourite foods. I was pleased that Jonathan ate a few sandwiches and sat with the other members for a short while to eat. I encouraged them to sit together and to talk about the foods they liked at the party. I observed that after eating they wanted to carry on with singing and using the instruments. A happy atmosphere had been created where I knew that they were all enjoying the social occasion. I made sure that the motivation and fun continued until the finishing time, then they had a surprise present to take home. The preparation and effort that I had put into the planning was all worthwhile! Seeing how Jonathan and the others coped enjoying themselves, as I had arranged the party to suit their needs, was wonderful progress and it made me determined to go forward with my vision for the group.

Continuing to work with Jonathan on all his skills (as we had been doing over the years) was helping him in his development, and I knew it would be ongoing. Music and singing were also proving to be an amazing interest which

Jonathan enjoyed; it was having wonderfully positive benefits to his confidence, social and communication skills, which were difficult for him as he was approaching twenty-two years old. Something inside of me made me feel that singing might be *the* way in which I could help Jonathan with his speech. He was beginning to sing his songs and follow the lyrics more confidently but still had limited speech in his everyday life. This was a part of his autism which I wanted to learn about, and I aimed to expand his music interest with time.

Having a small group to help with socialising was wonderful. I knew that I had to carry on and to continue to fund it myself until I could receive any additional funding. The experience of music, singing, playing musical instruments, and the noticeable effects it was having on Jonathan and myself urged me to want to learn more in order to develop my group that would help people with autism and learning disabilities.

Jonathan's choice in music was expanding and he was able to look for the lyrics to the songs in order to copy them. He had accrued several folders by now where his lyrics were numbered and indexed. I encouraged him to write them himself, to help him with his reading and writing. Additionally, he was using the computer to find the lyrics. He took his folders to the music group each week and put the sheets of paper on the music stand to follow the lyrics when singing. The other members wanted to know what he was doing and I explained what they were. I realised that it would be helpful for them if each member had a folder with their lyrics to follow because to sing along, they needed to know the lyrics, and very often they didn't! I put the suggestion to their support workers, I explained how it would be of great benefit to their reading skills and would enable them to enjoy the songs they wanted to sing along to. To my surprise, they seemed interested, and informed me that they would see what they could do. I felt confident that if the members had the lyrics to their songs, they would be able to sing along, which would help them to enjoy their music.

A few weeks went by and the members hadn't brought their folders. I asked their support workers about it, and was told the support workers hadn't had time. Not wanting to cause any issues, and feeling frustrated by their lack of interest, there was nothing more to be said! I felt sorry for those they were supposed to be supporting, and somewhat despondent, after all the time and effort I was devoting to the group voluntarily. I knew the members *could* get so much more from the music sessions if only they were given more support.

I supported Jonathan in any way possible. Feelings of doubting myself started to dominate my thoughts. I questioned what I was trying to achieve.

The lack of motivation from support workers was difficult for me to accept but prepared to tolerate; if only they would try and help those who they were supporting. Their attitude was affecting *my* mental health which I could not let happen anymore. I was giving my time voluntarily and funding the group myself, which was a financial struggle, but I was willing to do to help my son and others.

Always looking for other activities which could help Jonathan to progress, I was thinking about music session ideas that could encourage interaction. I decided to look for dance groups that might be of help to Jonathan and that we could introduce to our music group. I came across a line dancing group which met locally each week. Knowing nothing about line dancing, after making enquiries and talking with the teacher about Jonathan's autism, he reassured me that the group was small and friendly, and that we would be made welcome to go along and to see if it was for us.

After talking to Jonathan about going to a dance group, he did seem willing to try, which I was so pleased about. I was thinking about his coordination and movement; and in time wanted to show the members in our group what he was learning, thinking it may encourage them to try some dance movements.

The day of our dancing group arrived and I was a little nervous, as Jonathan was too. When we got to the group the others made us feel welcome, which was a lovely surprise. The teacher took time to show us the basic movements of each dance and I was amazed how quickly Jonathan had remembered the sequence of each dance! Line dancing did not require a partner, which was the main reason I had chosen that group; part of his autism meant he did not want anyone too close. He remembered each movement and steps he was following as the teacher demonstrated. I was so pleased to see how Jonathan was progressing and socialising in an environment where he could join in and feel confident.

He was dancing along with others, which was wonderful progress!

The line dancing classes suited Jonathan and he was enjoying taking part. I could see his progress, as he remembered each dance.

With their repetition and sequence, he coped well with it, and I felt that it was part of his autism. I was so pleased to see his coordination skills were developing, amazed at his ability to remember each dance; even if the teacher changed the music which was usually played to a certain dance. Jonathan remembered the sequence of the dance!

Having the experience of a new activity of dancing. I was continuing to learn about my son's autism and how it affected him. It also gave me ideas on how to develop the music group, by introducing simple dance steps which I felt that members could manage.

As we learnt and felt confident with several dance sequences, I encouraged Jonathan to show the others of our music group that which we had learnt, and encouraged them to join in. I was very surprised that they wanted to try some simple steps with us. Again, it was something I wanted to expand upon in order to help the group work together, and to improve upon their coordination skills.

I was hoping that the support workers would play a more active role, but to my disappointment, they showed little interest. Not wanting to jeopardise the position of those members who were really enjoying the music group from coming to us, I had to accept that any progress made would be from the motivation I put into the group.

I began to understand that our members liked different songs and dance movements. I was becoming more aware of the importance of music for autistic people. It was giving me various ideas on how I wanted the group to develop. The need to apply for funding made me determined to search for where I could possibly obtain any, to enable me to purchase musical equipment. I wanted to give our members the opportunity to explore music in ways that suited their needs. I needed room hire funding to be able to offer that opportunity on a regular basis, without the financial pressure on myself. I started to search for grants in the hope that my vision would be appreciated and understood and considered worthy of support.

Jonathan was continuing to make progress as we worked on his sensory, coordination, reading, writing and self-care skills. His cooking skills were improving slowly too. His appetite was starting to change a little, as was his willingness to try different foods. His mental wellbeing and behaviour were becoming calmer, and I felt that the herbal medicine which he had been continuing to take was helping lessen his stress. This meant that he was becoming more confident in trying out new activities. Music was having a wonderful result upon his confidence. Building friendships and learning teamwork in an environment he and the other members felt happy in was proving that I *had* to go forward in expanding my vision for the group.

Each week at our music group I could see how Jonathan and the other members were enjoying their time together. I would encourage Jonathan to demonstrate a few line dancing steps, and was so pleased that the others wanted to try them with us.

As usual, the support workers did not want to actively join in (which was very frustrating) but I tried to focus on the goal that I was trying to achieve with the members. The lack of motivation from support workers worried me, and I wondered how I could develop the group for those people who needed the opportunity of having somewhere to go and socialise in a happy, safe, environment. Whenever a new person joined, I was always hopeful that the workers would be different and would be interested in the person they were supposed to be supporting; that they would join in and want to motivate that person.

To my disappointment, some members were not able to continue being with us each week, or in other words, their support workers did not want to bring them! I felt this was an issue which needed looking into by social services, but I did not have the time to take that on. It was a more complex issue than just a lack of motivation from support workers!

I continued to fill out many applications for funding; only to be turned down because of the small number of people I could offer the opportunity to. This was very frustrating as I had explained each time that the need for a small group was so important to people with autism in order for them to be able to cope with different people and sounds.

I was becoming despondent through having to fund the group myself.

This was a financial struggle but I knew that it was helping Jonathan and the other members. I was concerned about how long that I would be able to continue funding it, and to achieve my vision of developing it without some financial help.

The summer was approaching, as was Jonathan's birthday. The Christmas party had been successful and my thoughts turned to the possibility of having a birthday party for him; combining music, and introducing a little difference, so that Jonathan and the other members could enjoy themselves in a special occasion for Jonathan to remember. We hadn't been able to celebrate his birthday over the years in a way adults of his age—now approaching twenty-three years old—without autism probably would, by having parties with friends and relatives, as Jonathan would not be able to cope with large groups. By keeping it small in number, as I did with the Christmas party, I felt that Jonathan and the other members would feel happy. They would not feel threatened!

I talked to Jonathan about the idea of having a birthday party with the music group. He started to accept that it would be a special day for him with his friends at the music group. I put the idea to the other members and their support workers about a date. They all seemed happy about the idea. I was able to set a date that suited everyone and was close to Jonathan's birthday. It would also give me time to plan and juggle my finances to pay for it. I felt that it was important to Jonathan's development to be able to socialise, and to be able to acknowledge special occasions like his birthday, even if he didn't fully understand how old he would be. To him it was his birthday, which meant it was a special day for him! I continued to plan for the birthday party and encourage the members each week to enjoy each music group session, while learning all the time about each member, including their likes and dislikes. This enabled me to structure each music session by taking into consideration all those issues.

It didn't really affect me too much that any support workers who were there did not show any motivation towards those that they were supposed to be supporting. It made me more determined to cultivate the group in a way which I felt was appropriate to suit the members' needs.

My thoughts turned to funding and being able to continue to develop the music group. I was being turned down by local grant sources. I decided to try for a lottery grant. Even though I felt that it was an impossible task, something inside me made me feel there was a chance. After being turned down by local funders, I had nothing to lose by applying to the lottery.

After making enquiries about the acceptance rules in order to apply for a grant, I had to get over the obstacle of opening a bank account. Although I had no money, and just a name for my group, having a bank account was essential in order to support my application. After trying several banks and being turned down, I finally found a bank which was willing to give a non-profit, voluntary organisation an account. I completed the necessary documentation to support my application for a lottery grant. The application form for such a grant was lengthy. It enabled me to describe the group and the benefits I was hoping to achieve, and the reasons why a small group was so important for autistic people. This helped me to explain my vision and how I felt it could help my son and others who had similar disabilities. I knew the completed application was to take six months before a decision was made. Having completed the application and posted it, my thoughts were now on Jonathan's birthday party.

When the day arrived of the party, Jonathan and the other members knew it was his special day. They gave him birthday cards and presents which made him feel special. We kept to the structure of our usual music session but added different songs and sang 'Happy Birthday' to Jonathan, who blew out candles on his cake. We moved away a little from the routine in a way they were able to cope with. I knew routine and structure were so important to autistic people; being able to cope with small changes would help them to be able to experience so much more.

Jonathan and the other members were showing how their confidence was improving in being able to cope with changes to their routine, if they were prepared and knew what changes to expect. I had learnt so much from my son about his autism over the years. I felt confident and able to understand others and it gave me the awareness of how I wanted to develop the group.

Jonathan's twenty-third birthday party was a success; everyone enjoyed themselves. The social skills which had been building between members and the confidence they were gaining was amazing to see. I knew that the group had so much to offer and expand upon if I had the funding to do so. I had to put the lottery application to the back of my thoughts after posting it, and stay focused on what I was trying to achieve with Jonathan; all of the skills we had been working on to help in his development, which were ongoing and important for him. Although line dancing was a new activity for Jonathan too, it also helped our music group. I was always looking for other experiences which could help his development.

I had to call into our local wood yard to find out the cost of a piece of wood to repair a door at home. In the reception office I saw some wonderful carved statues of animals. I asked the person at the desk who had made them. She told me of one of the workers who went to a local wood carving group. I enquired about the details, those she was happy to give me. My thoughts were to find out if it could be something Jonathan would be able to try, not expecting him of course to produce anything like I saw in the office of the wood yard, but to at least try.

I was not putting any limitations on my son having as many opportunities as possible, however impossible they may be understood by others.

I phoned the person who ran the wood carving group, and described Jonathan's autism, his skills in using tools at the heritage railway, and his ability to remember what he is shown to do. The main concerns of the person who ran the group was the ability and safety of Jonathan and him being able to use the different tools to do wood carving. I explained that I would be supporting him, and that I would know what words to use to help Jonathan understand that which he needed to.

I appreciated those concerns regarding safety issues, but I felt after seeing what was involved that I would know if it would benefit Jonathan, if he was given the opportunity to try. To my surprise, Jonathan was given the opportunity to join the small wood carving group. The people were friendly and accepted Jonathan and me (for which I was so pleased); another opportunity for Jonathan's sake! The other members were very talented at wood carving; they had been going to the group for many years. The person who ran the group who was called Mike, was an amazingly talented wood carver. I did doubt myself about joining the group knowing that I would never be able to learn those skills, and I wasn't sure if Jonathan would be able to do wood carving.

On the first visit Jonathan was given a piece of wood and a stencil of a leaf to draw around. This was an exercise which all new people started to work on. I observed as Jonathan was being instructed and was so pleased that he was following what he was expected to do. After drawing the leaf on the piece of wood, Jonathan had to use a small tool to cut away the wood from around the leaf. After reminding Jonathan of the safety issues on using the tools, Mike felt confident that Jonathan could carry on by himself whilst he attended to the others. I watched Jonathan as he used the tools and was amazed at how quickly he was able to carve away the wood to form the leaf.

His hand-eye coordination was wonderful to see. It was a completely different skill from the use of heavy railway tools and yet he was enjoying this new activity with confidence. After an hour or so, Jonathan had formed the leaf from the piece of wood. This surprised Mike and he informed me that it usually took new members three or four weeks to do what Jonathan had done in an hour; each session was three hours long! I felt that Jonathan had proved himself, and that helped Mike to overcome his concerns about safety and Jonathan's ability to use the tools. It made me realise that my son had so much more to be developed. I was pleased that he had been given the opportunity to join the small, very talented, wood carving group.

It was a calm environment with low background music playing. Each week a member would make tea or coffee, speak to Jonathan about his work, and how well he was doing.

They were accepting him, which was so important for us both. When I decided to take my turn at making the drinks, Jonathan would come round with me and write down each person's name and what drink they wanted. It helped him to get to know their names and to build up his confidence in being part of that group. I was also showing others that autistic people *can* achieve, given the opportunity and respect. Jonathan would wash the cups and tidy the kitchen area (as was expected of everyone in the group); I was encouraging his independence skills in a different environment, and so pleased that he felt happy too about doing it.

As Mike was seeing how well Jonathan was able to use the tools and had finished the leaf with very detailed leaf patterns, he was able to expand his skills to try other objects to carve. I explained that Jonathan liked trains, not knowing if it was possible for him to do one. Mike got a book to show Jonathan which had some trains in, but they were not the ones he liked. I suggested that Jonathan could bring in one to show Mike which train he would like to try. Jonathan seemed very happy about carving a train. The following week Jonathan chose a picture of The Rocket, the first steam train built by George Stevenson. Mike was surprised at Jonathan's choice and wasn't sure how it could be done as he had never been asked by anyone before to do a train.

I suggested that Jonathan could draw it as he had amazing hand-eye coordination for detail. After giving Jonathan some paper and pencils to draw The Rocket (which he did with precise detail) Mike could work on the size and figure out which wood to use, as a cutting tool would be needed for the wheels and other parts. Mike was so amazed at the drawing of the train, done in such a short time. He wanted to show the other members what Jonathan had drawn. I encouraged Jonathan to take his drawing round to show each member. They were surprised at the detail and praised Jonathan on his skills. I was so pleased that Jonathan was raising awareness and understanding of the talents autistic people have. The new skills he was learning at wood carving continued to amaze me. It proved that by giving Jonathan opportunities to learn, he could achieve much more. I would not put limitations on him to explore different opportunities to progress.

I felt that the other members were starting to understand more about Jonathan and were less fearful of talking to him. As Jonathan started on the carving of The Rocket, it was a topic of conversation for the group each week. Mike had confidence in Jonathan's skills in using various tools after he'd been shown how to use them. He knew that he could leave him to get on with carving. As I was observing Jonathan and trying to be sociable with the other members, I started by talking about the other things which he was doing such as with the music group. I encouraged Jonathan to say which songs he liked, and the instruments he enjoyed playing. I wanted to expand the understanding of people with autism. I appreciated that we were in a group of extremely talented wood carvers, but I still felt that it was important for them to understand that other skills and talents were beneficial too. Mike encouraged me to have a try at wood carving a leaf, just as Jonathan had done so well. He understood that I was supporting Jonathan but felt that it would be helpful for me to try for myself as Jonathan had settled into the group, and knew what he was doing on his own project. It wasn't until I began to carve a leaf that I realised how difficult it was to use the tools to make each accurate cutting of the wood. Although I had watched Jonathan when he started his project, I did not fully appreciate those skills which were needed. This made me even more aware of the progress and talent my son had.

Having the wonderful opportunity to be part of the wood carving group, seeing Jonathan progress in his project with The Rocket train, I felt that there was so much more Jonathan could show others and myself of his ability to learn.

With the music group, line dancing classes, and wood carving, I felt that Jonathan was developing his social and coordination skills, which I had been working on over the years. He was proving that it was needed as part of his development. To be at the stage he was at this point in time. I was happy for him and never once regretted putting in all that time and effort over his life. To see him improve was just a miracle! And I am so pleased, as his mother, to be continuing to learn about my son's autism and how it affects his daily life; to find as many opportunities as possible to bring out his talents and skills.

The music group was developing slowly each week. The members were becoming more confident with each other. I continued to encourage teamwork and social skills by greeting each other, and by trying to encourage eye contact. I felt that the music group and wood carving group were helping Jonathan to progress his development. This was the confirmation for me that I was doing the best I could to give my son a quality of life where he was happy and safe in environments which suited his needs, while also helping others (as in the music group). He was raising awareness of autism and the wonderful skills autistic people can have if given the opportunity.

As always, the financial costs of any activities I found for my son were a concern. I wanted to give him every opportunity that I could but I knew that balancing the costs was difficult. I was reaching the stage where I would have to choose between paying for the music group room hire or attending the wood carving group. I felt down and depressed because I knew that both groups were helping Jonathan (and others too), but I couldn't continue payment for both.

It had been a few months since I had posted the lottery application, with no acknowledgement! This started to make me feel despondent and thoughts that my vision of how I wanted to develop the small group to suit the needs of autistic people was a waste of time. It would not be understood! The wood carving group was helping Jonathan to make an object that he could take home and keep. Both activities had beneficial outcomes, but I was getting closer to having to make a choice on which one I could afford to carry on with.

I explained my problem to the wood carving teacher Mike, who was very understanding and offered me a reduced rate. I was supporting Jonathan and could not be taking up anyone's place. I was pleased and appreciated his help so that Jonathan could continue to be part of the group. It also enabled me to continue funding the music group. With the financial stress eased, I could enjoy focusing on both groups. The members at the wood carving group wanted to know more about our music group. To help Jonathan with his social and communication skills, they would ask him about the songs he liked to sing, and involved him in conversation.

Jonathan was making wonderful progress with his carving of the train. He wanted to finish it before the group stopped for Christmas, which was not far away.

I had been planning the Christmas party, and Jonathan was happy to talk about it to the members of the wood carving group. He wanted to show his train to the music group. He was working very hard to finish his train in time, and I could see the concentration he had each week in order to finish it. The music playing in the background was of Christmas songs; when Jonathan heard those he liked, he stopped what he was doing to listen to the song and tell the group that it was what he sang at music group. His confidence and speech were improving; I had waited for many years to see it, always hoping for progress. For me, his mother, to see it now was a miracle.

The train was finished in time for Christmas! Mike was so pleased in the manner which Jonathan had completed it, as were the other members, who could appreciate the skill Jonathan was showing. After wishing everyone a Happy Christmas and looking forward to starting again in the new year, Jonathan could take his train to show the members of our music group. I could see how he felt a sense of achievement and wanted to show others whom he had built friendships with. Seeing the progress which had taken many years to achieve made it all worthwhile. I knew that more progress would be made in the future.

The Christmas party was nearing! All the planning I had put into it in order to make it a happy occasion for Jonathan and the others made me feel happy that I was able to get through another year, and that they were looking forward to celebrating Christmas in a way which suited their needs.

I managed to purchase small gifts for everyone, and foods they liked; keeping to a structure they knew but varying it a little. I was confident that it would be a success.

On the day of the party, I was busy making sure that I had everything I needed to take to the hall. The post was earlier than usual; I noticed an envelope with the Lottery logo on it. I felt very nervous, not knowing whether to open it or not.

I had prepared myself over the months that the application would be turned down. I was looking forward to the Christmas party and making it a happy occasion for everyone. I did not want the news, if it was a rejection, to affect my feelings at the party and letting the members down. I decided to open the letter. When I read the first line, 'Congratulations on your application'. I could not believe what I was reading! It took several minutes to compose my feelings of absolute *joy*, not for myself, but knowing that I could continue the group and expand the opportunity to explore a variety of musical instruments. I had another idea I'd wanted to try, should I get this funding. I had costed it out but I hadn't mentioned it to Jonathan or anyone else so as not to disappoint them. I wanted to have an art group to help Jonathan and others enjoy being creative. I was aware of Jonathan's skill at drawing and I felt that if he could socialise with others doing another activity which they enjoyed, it would help further develop his confidence and communication skills and building of friendships.

The music group members were getting on with each other, and they were happy with the structure of the group. I was hoping they would want to try art too. I decided to have leaflets printed to offer the opportunity to others who wanted to join us. Both groups would be small in numbers. I was so relieved that the financial strain had been lifted off my shoulders and was excited about developing the groups, knowing that I had been given the opportunity to realise my vision of helping autistic people!

Uniquely Me & U was going forward and being recognised as a worthwhile project for the community.

At the end of the successful party, I mentioned to the support workers about having an art group as well as music in the new year, and if they thought those people whom they supported would like to try it. Details would be given as soon as I had sorted out a day and time. I needed to know if they wanted to come, as I was going to have leaflets distributed in various places to offer the opportunity to others.

Over the Christmas break I talked to Jonathan about drawing, painting and having others to join us at the hall on another day. He seemed to accept the idea. He liked going to the wood carving group, and I suggested that he could paint his train and leaf which he had made at the art group and show it to the other members. I wasn't sure if anyone from the music group would come, or if the others would be interested, but I wanted to try. I felt it was the right way to go to help my son and I felt confident that others would join us in time.

There was no rush to start an art group and I did not want to use the funding without careful thought as to what I would be purchasing. I felt so grateful to be able to offer the activities for the coming year, and I was going to take it all steadily.

When enquiring at the hall if another day was available to hire for an art group. I was informed that there were no other days available, as it was fully booked. This meant trying to find another room which was affordable within the grant which I had applied for from the Lottery money. After many phone calls about room hire and cost, most were too expensive! When I was walking through the local town to look at a music equipment shop, I noticed a large poster advertisement for a local room to hire. After taking the details and walking to find out where it was, I was pleasantly surprised at the location; a bus stop was close. I phoned to ask about room hire costs, and after explaining to the person who dealt with hiring about my group, he offered an affordable cost, should it be suitable for the needs of the people who would be using it. After going to look at the room and talking to Jonathan about doing art at the 'new room'. I wanted to see how he reacted, as autistic people find it difficult to go into different environments. This I understood and accepted!

When we were shown the room, kitchen, toilets and car park (which all seemed very suitable and pleasant) Jonathan showed himself to be settled. We walked around, and it felt right for the groups to take place there. After confirming that I would hire the room but would have to inform others that we were moving the group, I would phone to advise when the group would start.

When I left the new room, I felt it was an exciting phase for Jonathan and I; with the hope of meeting others who would help to develop Uniquely Me & U.

After letting the support workers know the music group would be moving to another room locally, I informed them they would still be able to bring members, and that it was where our art group would be too. I decided that it would be better if we did not go back to the old hall but make a fresh start at the new room.

The Christmas break would help the group accept somewhere new.

I purchased some musical instruments to begin with (I decided to introduce others gradually) after I had learnt more about just what musical instruments the members would like. Jonathan came to the shop with me to look at all the various instruments, which the assistant was happy to show us, encouraging Jonathan to try any that he liked. I explained to the assistant I wanted instruments which would be easy for our members to play. As our group evolved, I would be aware of what other instruments may be beneficial to purchase. When we were about to leave Jonathan went to look at a keyboard at the back of the shop. I had noticed it when we first went into the shop but I did not think that it would be an instrument which the group members would be ready for. The assistant encouraged him to play it; to my surprise Jonathan liked the sounds as he pressed various keys in a careful gentle way. Due to the cost, he had not had the opportunity to have a keyboard before. I had to admit to myself that I thought being able to play a keyboard would be too difficult for Jonathan, and yet he was showing a keen interest in the sounds of a keyboard. The assistant offered to sell it at a reduced price as it was for a group which was helping disabled people. I reminded myself about not putting limitations on my son, and how he could easily prove to me how wrong I was in thinking that it might be too difficult for him to play. I agreed to buy the keyboard for our music group with the intention of learning to play it myself so that I could, in turn, help our members who were interested too.

The day arrived of the first music group of Uniquely Me & U, with Jonathan and another member who was part of the group when we met at the hall. Being at a new room did make them a little nervous. We had to find out the best places to put the musical equipment which suited them; by having the same routine and structure as they were used to, helped them to settle down and to enjoy their music. I set up the keyboard and encouraged Jonathan to play some sounds, hoping the other member would also want to try it, along with the other instruments I had purchased. It took time and encouragement for them to explore the new instruments which I completely understood and accepted. Every step had to be at their own pace. The first session was a little difficult and strange for the members, but I felt confident that after that day, things would become easier for them. They would have routine and structure while having fun and being able to express themselves through music, which they had chosen and felt happy with. I developed it gradually, with others who wanted to join us, keeping a calm, harmonious, atmosphere. This was very important for members to feel safe and secure, to be able to grow in confidence. I had learnt this over the years by understanding how Jonathan's autism affected him in different environments. I knew which environment was needed for him and for others with similar disabilities. Having the funding to create that environment and giving those people somewhere to go and to socialise, to make friends, and be happy was a wonderful opportunity for me too, to continue learning how I could help my son and others.

Over the weeks I received enquiries from parents and support workers about both groups. I had a start date for the art group. I decided to call it a 'creative art' group, as I wanted members to choose what they decided to do, and be encouraged to explore art and to express themselves through their own ideas. I had purchased a variety of art materials to begin the group and would add more as the members progressed. At the start it was Jonathan and another autistic person, with her mother who was supporting her. The mother knew it was important for her daughter to settle in her own time and I was also aware that Jonathan was anxious at having different people in the room too.

I encouraged Jonathan to draw his trains or whatever he would choose, and to show the new member. It was a calm, quiet atmosphere; one that helped us all to get used to each other.

I felt so pleased to meet another mother who was also motivated in wanting to help her daughter, and knew it was important for her to be able to make friends in an environment which suited her needs. I explained that the group would be small, with only five or six people, which the mother appreciated was important. Over the weeks, Jonathan and the new member were accepting each other. I was becoming more aware of the autistic traits of the new member and understanding how to help her interact a little each week with Jonathan. This is what I had the aims and hopes for; I wanted to build and develop a social group where they could express themselves through art.

Jonathan was becoming more confident and would help to set out the tables, chairs, materials for the art group, and music equipment on the day we had music. He was showing initiative and a sense of responsibility to help the other members who were not able to do that. In such a short time of forming the creative art group and music group, I could see that wonderful progress Jonathan was making, and how other members were interacting with each other in small ways, by cooperating, taking turns, listening to songs others had chosen, showing one another their creative art. Each group was developing slowly, which was important, and it was proving to be beneficial for improving their confidence; not only Jonathan's, but the other members' also.

When Jonathan went back to the wood carving group. I would encourage him to tell the group what he was doing in the art or music group. It was letting others know how people with autism and learning disabilities could achieve, if they were given the opportunity and respect.

I felt it was helping to raise awareness for people who had no experience or contact with anyone like Jonathan or our group members. The wood carving group was gaining an understanding and respect for Jonathan and the skills he was showing. I had an idea for Jonathan to take his finished wood carvings to the art group to paint, and to show the others just what he had achieved. He liked that idea very much. It meant that he was connecting his groups, and he could have a topic of conversation to encourage his communication skills, which had always been my aim.

As I was getting more interest from people to join in both of the groups, I felt excited that my hopes and vision of having a happy and safe environment where Jonathan and others could go and socialize, while enjoying activities they liked and building friendships were finally coming true. It was something I did not think would ever happen, after all the years of being disappointed at not being able to find suitable groups for Jonathan and living an isolated life, not being able to be part of his community. I was determined to make sure that this opportunity I had, which was considered a worthwhile project to fund, would be a success in helping my son and others who may wish to join us.

We had two new members who wanted to join our creative art group. After talking to the parents of both people, I tried to find out about their disabilities so that I could help them as much as possible to enjoy the group. The two new members would not have a support worker with them as they were able to make their own way to the group. I was looking forward to meeting them. I had prepared Jonathan and the other member about the new people who would be joining us.

Preparation and planning I felt was important when doing anything different or not part of the group's normal routine. Our new members were verbal and able to be encouraged to interact within the group. I was learning about different disabilities and how they affected people.

Although their communication skills were clearer than Jonathan's and the other member's, I was aware how limited their understanding was when I asked them questions. It was wonderful that they were able to come to the group independently and to settle in so quickly. I would spend some time with each member, finding out about their creative art, which colours they liked, if they liked to use pencils, paints or other art materials we had. After talking to each member, I would then encourage each of them to get up from their table and to go over to the other members to show them what they were drawing, painting or making. I knew autistic people and anyone with learning disabilities find it very difficult to make eye contact or to be able to make conversation within a group. Because our group was small, it was giving them the confidence as they got to know each other, learning about interests the members had by talking about their creative art. Jonathan liked trains, others liked animals, sea, sand, and flowers. There was so much to learn about each member through art.

This I found amazing, and it was giving me the opportunity to find other ways to keep developing the group.

In the music group we had new members join who came with their support workers. I explained how our group was structured. When everyone took turns to sing or to listen to their own songs. Jonathan would write down the name of the member and chosen song so that everyone knew whose turn it was next.

I asked the support workers to encourage their member to try the musical instruments if they felt happy to do so. With each new member I had to rely upon the support worker to encourage that person to settle in as I did not want to cause them to be anxious. When I thought that the time was right to interact with that new member, I would sing along to their song or encourage them to do some simple dance movements. At times, if the support workers showed little motivation and left it to me, I would encourage the member to interact with the group members to get their reactions, as I felt that otherwise they would be left to just sit and watch the others, which I did not think was helping them to feel part of the group. I was gaining confidence with how I wanted to further develop each group by meeting others with similar issues as Jonathan, along with people with different disabilities. They all were responding in a positive way, enjoying the creative art and music group, because it was an environment which suited their needs. Groups were small and the sessions were calm, structured and harmonious; where they felt safe and happy to express themselves without judgement.

The progress the members were making was proving how important opportunity was for my son. He could not go out on his own to socialise or build friendships, as with those who joined us. Forming Uniquely Me & U was giving them their own social groups and helping them to improve their skills. I felt that the support workers did not understand my aims and hopes for each group. I was doing it voluntarily, with funding, and they expected me to do the motivating and encouraging! This disappointed me. I knew that all the members could achieve so much more if everyone worked together. I tried not to think about it too much, and to stay focused on what I wanted for the members. I could see how much Jonathan was improving by having the groups each week, and that made all the time and effort that I was putting into the groups worthwhile.

Jonathan's life was structured, with various opportunities for him to keep improving his many skills. Always looking for new ideas, experiences which might help, I saw an advertisement in our local newspaper for volunteers to help a group which provided disabled people with communication aids which gave information about the local area, and poetry, sports news etc. Not knowing what was involved or needed to be done, I made enquiries and spoke to the organiser, who explained what they did.

After explaining Jonathan's autism and his brilliant memory, I felt that he would be able to help, with me supporting him. The organiser was happy for us to go along and see if it was something Jonathan would like. I talked to Jonathan about it, trying to get across as best I could what he would be doing with me helping him.

When we went to see the group and what they did, it seemed very interesting. I was hopeful that it could be beneficial for Jonathan, as one of the tasks involved speaking into a microphone to give sports results. Jonathan would not understand what they meant, but it would encourage his speech. I knew that he was able to read the words and numbers, maybe not as confidently as someone without communication difficulties, but I felt strongly that he could, with help, improve, and be helping others too. The readings were recorded and put onto a memory stick along with various other information. Each member of the group had their own topic which they recorded. The person who read poetry and historical items was a kind and considerate man and got along with Jonathan and me. His name was John, and he straight away understood why I had taken Jonathan to the group to help them. He was willing to help

Jonathan with his speech for recording. I was so pleased to have met someone who accepted my son for who he was.

A few weeks later John was showing us what had to be done to prepare papers for recording. Some of the other members did not seem to be happy about John showing my son anything. I tried to settle into the group and explain Jonathan's autism, but I felt that they did not want us to be there. After talking to John about it, he was disappointed in the way in which we were treated and understood why we could not stop there. I thanked him for his kindness but the attitude of the other group members was something we had experienced for many years.

I explained about the voluntary groups I was running and he was so happy about it. Wanting to know more about them, he said that he had worked with disabled people some years ago, and he had helped to set up a residential home for them. He had had a career in the RAF, enjoyed art and music, and offered his help at the groups as a volunteer. Being a quiet, calm person, I knew that he would be accepted by the members. I would certainly appreciate help and support to enable the group's development and to give the members every opportunity to progress, which I was always striving to do.

I was very disappointed with having to leave a group which I felt could have been beneficial for Jonathan. The attitude of those people who would not accept my son because of his autism was hurtful to me, and had started to affect Jonathan too, as he was sensitive to atmospheres and negative feelings from others. It would not have worked out. We had experienced that kind of prejudice on many occasions over the years, and it was still upsetting that society had not gained any understanding of autism, especially from a group which was supposed to be helping other disabled people. I realised that as recording was involved, certain people felt more important and capable than others to have their voices recorded. Having an autistic person who was not yet verbally competent would not be accepted in their group.

This was another harsh experience which I had to accept and try to put to the back of my mind. I knew how important it was to ensure that everyone who came to our groups were made to feel welcome and accepted.

John came to both the art and music group to help and to encourage our members, and to make any suggestions which could further develop their skills. Having someone who understood my aims and outcomes for the members was a wonderful help to me; this I appreciated very much. I could see how Jonathan and the others were progressing, as they were choosing to use different art materials. Some preferred painting, others drawing or making things from quick-drying clay.

I was always finding new ideas to help with their dexterity, coordination and expression, together with continuing to encourage their social skills and interaction. In music, Jonathan was improving in his choice of songs and being able to read the lyrics.

I was so pleased, as I knew that singing would help his speech. The members were confident in playing different instruments, making sounds they enjoyed. I explained to the support workers that if their members could have the lyrics to the songs they liked, it would help them to sing along and enjoy their music more. I had been hoping for their cooperation in order to give members the opportunity to achieve. I was disappointed when I was informed that reading would be difficult for the members. Although the members were close in age to Jonathan or older, it did not occur to me that they hadn't been taught to read. All had been through the education system except for Jonathan; this made me realise that the decision I had made to take my son out of the system, and to do what I thought would help him was the right way for Jonathan.

I had to accept that the idea of members being capable of singing the lyrics was not going to happen. I had to focus on ways to help them to enjoy their music.

Jonathan was becoming more interested in playing the keyboard and making his own sounds. When other members chose to have a go, they liked pressing all the keys and finding sounds which they liked, but they enjoyed the other instruments more, like the xylophone or tambourines. The members enjoyed music in their own way and encouraged one another in their different choice of songs and instruments they liked to use. They were working together as a group, where they could express themselves without anyone judging them.

I felt that Jonathan was now ready to be shown the basics of playing the keyboard, and if that were possible, then hopefully in time he could show the other members who wanted to try. Again, I was thinking of teamwork, cooperation and other social skills by giving the opportunity to achieve. I decided to look for a music teacher who was able to show Jonathan the basics of playing the keyboard. I made several enquiries and was turned down because of Jonathan's autism; the teachers I spoke to had no experience in working with an autistic person and were not willing to try. I was disappointed with the lack of understanding about autism and the skills autistic people have that are not recognised until they are given opportunities to develop them. I was not going to give up looking for a teacher, but I knew it would take time to find one.

When going to the musical instrument shop to purchase more items, I mentioned to the assistant that I was having difficulty in finding a music teacher to help Jonathan with playing the keyboard because of his autism. The assistant gave me the details of a teacher who was known very well in that shop and taught privately as well as in schools. After purchasing some instruments, and thanking the assistant for the details, I felt optimistic that this person might help. I contacted the teacher and explained Jonathan's autism, his very good memory, and his willingness to listen and be shown. To my surprise the teacher, whose name was Chris, said that he hadn't worked with autistic adults or children but would try. He agreed to a time which suited Jonathan, on a day we were not going to the groups. I wanted Jonathan to have the opportunity to see if he could learn to play simple tunes, then go on to help our group members to try and learn to play some tunes. The cost of private lessons I felt that I could manage, as the pressure of funding the groups was now supported by the lottery grant, which was an enormous help.

Chris was a calm easy-going person, which helped Jonathan to accept him. I sat near to Jonathan to help him understand any of the instructions Chris was giving. I couldn't play the keyboard either, but I wanted to learn in order to help the group. Firstly, Chris put some letters on the keyboard in order to show Jonathan the basic keys he would start with: CDEFGAB. Chris asked Jonathan to say the letters out loud and was pleasantly surprised that he knew his alphabet. I had explained to Chris that Jonathan has learnt to read and write over the years and would remember that which he was shown.

After his first lesson learning about the keys and using his fingers to play the notes, I observed how quickly Jonathan was enjoying learning about the basic notes and playing them. Chris was surprised too, having been concerned before meeting Jonathan that he would not be able to teach him. After Jonathan's first lesson, it was clear to us all that Jonathan had the ability to learn to play. I booked the next lesson, and I made the decision for Jonathan to have a lesson every fortnight, which I could manage financially. I felt that through singing, dancing and playing the keyboard (an instrument which Jonathan had chosen), music was having a wonderful effect on his mental health.

His confidence was improving, together with his social skills! I saw that with Chris, Jonathan listened to him, and interacted verbally when asked about letters and making the sounds of the scales. This was again a new experience for Jonathan and me, and I knew it could have amazing outcomes for Jonathan and the other members over time. I was beginning to understand how important music was for Jonathan, who once again was proving his ability to learn, if given the opportunity. It confirmed the belief I had in my son and the wonderful skills he had. I was determined to help him develop them! Chris was the right person to help Jonathan, although at times he needed guidance from me to find the right words when explaining something to him. Chris knew that Jonathan had the ability to learn to play the keyboard, which I was so pleased about.

In our music group, I encouraged Jonathan to help the other members who wanted to play the keyboard, to learn the letters CDEFGAB. By singing the sounds of the scales as a group, it was keeping it fun to learn something new. It was another experience I could encourage Jonathan to talk about at the wood carving group.

I continued to raise awareness of the skills and progress Jonathan was making, and helped our groups develop. By helping others learn new skills too, Jonathan was connecting his group; at wood carving, when he had finished an object, he would take it to the art group to paint, then take it back to the wood carving group to show them how he had painted it. I was helping him connect his activities, using this as a talking point and raising an awareness of his wider skills. Learning to play the keyboard was another topic of conversation for all of the groups. One or two members at the wood carving group could play a piano or keyboard, and appreciated how Jonathan was progressing in other skills.

This helped others to accept and understand how autistic people can, and are, capable of achieving if they are given the opportunity! That is after experiencing many years of prejudice and isolation from society's lack of understanding of autism.

I felt that Jonathan had a quality of life that I had worked so hard over the years to attain for him. Struggling through those difficult and lonely times with no support, with only the love and motivation to help my son. He had opportunities to socialise, progress and to achieve new skills. It was a miracle to see how he had progressed, and how caring he was towards others, wanting to help the members who had become his friends.

He enjoyed his keyboard lessons, and Chris was building a good working relationship with Jonathan. He found different ways of helping Jonathan to follow music and to use both hands. This showed how his coordination skills were improving, as was his ability to follow music and understand the chords and notes. This was an amazing achievement for Jonathan, who really enjoyed learning to play the keyboard. I *knew* Chris was the right person to encourage Jonathan and would continue to bring out his musical skills.

The creative art group was developing in the way in which I had hoped. The members were happy and growing in confidence. They were willing to try different materials to create their own art! As each member progressed, I got to know more of their likes and dislikes. I had an idea for them to do a group topic to encourage their teamwork. Jonathan liked trains, another member liked animals, birds, flowers, dinosaurs. I suggested they create their own circus scene on a large canvas and to put whatever they wanted upon it. This idea was happily accepted. Each member knew what they were going to draw or paint for the canvas. It was going to take a number of weeks to complete! I felt it would encourage interaction, communication, social skills, and teamwork to create the canvas. The members were excited and happy, encouraging each other in their choice of that which they wanted to do for the circus scene.

In the music group, the members were enjoying doing some line dancing movement, and playing the musical instruments. Their choice of songs was expanding as they grew in confidence, teamwork, social skills, and respect for one another. This was wonderful to see. Jonathan would play the keyboard to show others what he was learning and was happy to let other members try to play, but they preferred other instruments! Both groups were having positive outcomes for Jonathan and the other members.

Seeing the wonderful progress, they were all making, it gave me the idea that the community should see that having a small group and encouraging each person to develop their skills at their own pace was proving to be beneficial in building confidence, social and communication skills. I wanted to do the same for the art group too, but it would have to be held on a different day, taking into consideration the needs of each group.

After talking about it to the members and getting their reactions, as I knew inviting strangers into the groups was difficult for people with autism and learning disabilities, I explained that it would be their parents, people whom they knew, together with others who wanted to see how well they were doing. To my surprise, their reactions were positive. They felt confident about showing the community what they were doing in both art and music. I decided to plan a date for each group, and to get some leaflets printed to display in the library, council office, churches and places where people may be interested in coming.

I also thought that I would ask our mayor of the town if he was available to come along and support our groups. To my pleasant surprise, the invitation was accepted!

The members were excited about the mayor coming to see them, together with other people in the community. Jonathan was progressing in his keyboard lessons, wanting to show the people what he was learning.

The circus scene canvas in the creative art group was developing well. I felt so happy for Jonathan and the other members. They had progressed enough to show the community and the mayor.

Uniquely Me & U was proving to have positive outcomes, because it took into consideration the members' needs and cultivated the groups *around* their needs.

There was a great deal of preparation for both groups for the planned dates. I was so proud and happy that both group members were confident about showing the public, and the mayor, just what they could do. It would prove to me that all the effort and time I had put into the groups was worthwhile; my aims and intentions were having positive outcomes both for Jonathan and other members!

When the day arrived for members of the community to be invited into the group, I was prepared for setbacks, as autistic people do not like strangers around them. To my surprise the members enjoyed showing their finished circus canvas and talking about what they had done to contribute to the scene. In music, the members sang their chosen songs and Jonathan played the keyboard. Both sessions went well, though not very well supported. The mayor, who himself was a local teacher, was very supportive of the progress they were making, and praised Jonathan for his keyboard skills.

We had a write-up in our local newspaper, and it was a wonderful treat for the members to see themselves in print.

It gave them the praise and confidence they had deserved so much. For me, it was an amazing achievement; our members had developed in their social and confidence skills; to have the public (whom they didn't know) come along and to see what they were capable of achieving, having been given the opportunity!

My thoughts turned to Jonathan and the way he was mastering the keyboard. I was beginning to understand that Jonathan enjoyed learning how to play music in a way I did not think he would be able to do. Chris was helping him to read the music notes, which improved Jonathan's confidence when playing. I felt that I should learn the basics of the keyboard to help our group members who wanted to play. I had the idea of purchasing another keyboard and leave the letters of the notes on the keys. Jonathan had progressed with his lessons and did not need them on his keyboard. Always having to be mindful of the costs, I decided to have fifteen minutes tuition after Jonathan had his lesson with Chris. After several lessons on the basics of playing the keyboard, I did purchase another one for the group. I put the letters on it and hoped it would encourage other members to try to play. I explained to the support workers about the basic notes, hoping that they would get involved and would encourage the members whom they were there to support. Sadly, this did not happen. I felt very disappointed that the members were not being encouraged as much as they should have been, and I was not able to give one-to-one attention to all the members, which I knew was needed if they were going to progress. It was very frustrating for me. I was aware that members had the ability to learn if they were supported and encouraged. I felt so pleased with the way Jonathan was progressing with his keyboard. Although he was willing to show others the basic notes, he could not understand why the members found it difficult to learn the letters CDEFGAB. That is the reason I decided that I needed to know more. I could not expect Jonathan (who had progressed beyond my hopes) to try and show others who were not encouraged outside of the group, how to play or learn the letters.

I was pleased with the development of the creative art and music group, and that the members themselves were making. Jonathan was improving in confidence as he felt a sense of belonging in the groups. I felt the other members did too. I had developed the groups slowly and taken into consideration each of the members' issues to help them to feel like an integral part of the group despite the lack of motivation from support workers, which was becoming more of a problem. I was motivated and encouraged each member of each group as much as possible, but I felt my vision, my hopes and aims were not properly understood by those whom I needed to work *with* me. I was giving up my time voluntarily to hold the groups because I could see the beneficial outcomes my son and the other members were experiencing, but I was aware of the lack of expectation of disabled people from those that were supposed to be encouraging them. I felt that this was an issue that needed to be addressed. I decided to keep a journal of the problems that occurred each week due to the lack of encouragement from the support workers. I started to think that I may be expecting too much from them and doubting myself and the reasons why I was running the groups. I knew I had made the right decision not to have any more support workers for my son, due to the lack of training and their limited understanding of autism.

I tried to stay focused on my aims and hopes for the groups; these were helping Jonathan and others who had joined us. Jonathan was making undreamed-of progress in his keyboard skills. Chris, his teacher, was appreciating the ability Jonathan had to learn as time passed.

My keyboard lessons were at the basic level, but enough to help members who wanted to try and play. Often Jonathan just wanted to get a feel for the keyboard and played different notes of the sounds he liked, knowing which notes he preferred. I now understood just how music was helping him in a completely different way, and I wanted to explore the subject more deeply.

Chris asked if Jonathan would like to take part in a music concert which he held every year for his students. I was very pleased that he had considered that Jonathan was progressing enough to take part, but was worried that his skills would not be at the level of his more talented students. Chris assured me that Jonathan would be able to play the pieces of music he had been confidently learning and would take his place like everyone else playing their chosen music. It would be a calm atmosphere and the audience respected that the students needed them to quietly listen and enjoy the music. Chris felt that Jonathan would be able to cope as he would be focusing on his music.

The date was set for later in the year, which gave Jonathan time to learn the music he would be playing. It gave Jonathan the opportunity to show the other members what he had been learning at his birthday party in the summer. He was now approaching twenty-four years old and we would be celebrating other members' birthdays too. I always made sure that the birthdays of all our members were special, and I encouraged everyone in their social skills in order to enjoy the atmosphere they felt happy and confident in. That was my intention, to make everyone feel part of the group and respected for who they were.

Time passed and the day of the concert arrived. Jonathan took his keyboard to set up at the room Chris had hired. I sat close to where he would be playing to help him settle and to encourage him. Chris informed me that he was holding the concert in aid of raising money for our group, Uniquely Me & U. He wanted me to give a short talk raising awareness of autism, talking about Jonathan and the progress he was making with his keyboard skills. I was nervous, but I felt so proud for my son that he was playing his music alongside the other students.

After my short talk, I was amazed at the wonderful support the audience showed towards Jonathan when he finished his music. I was so proud and happy for him that the audience appreciated his skills in playing the keyboard. My thoughts turned to the members of our music group, whom I felt were also capable of more, if only they had the support and encouragement. Sadly, I had to accept that all I could do was to make sure they enjoyed music as much as possible when they came to the group. I realised my son was able to learn so much more, and that was, and always would be my aim, hope and intention; to help him develop those skills.

We were approaching the end of the year for our groups, which the Lottery grant funded. It had been a busy but enjoyable time developing the groups. We'd invited the community and local mayor to see the progress members were making, Jonathan had taken part in a musical concert involving other talented students, and we had held birthday parties for Jonathan and other members. Now they were all looking forward to their Christmas party with joy. They knew what to expect and had formed friendships with each other. I was so pleased and grateful to have had the opportunity to develop the groups; to see the wonderful progress my son and the other members had made.

I was looking forward to the new year, as we had obtained funding to continue from the mayor's fund, Chris's music concert, the local council, and the local Masonic lodge.

I was thinking of the progress Jonathan was making in all of his various skills and his development over the years. Forming the creative art and music group had been the right way to go for him to help his communication and social skills, which had been affected greatly over his life due to the lack of opportunities which suited his needs. I knew I had to keep working on all of the issues in his development; his reading, writing, sensory, self-care and cooking skills, and trying to encourage him to expand his choices in food. That would be ongoing! I was aware that his social and communication skills were not improving as much as I had hoped because of his isolation, due to his autism, from the community.

Having the funding to form and develop Uniquely Me & U was a wonderful opportunity and had proved that it was the right way for Jonathan and those that joined us.

As my keyboard lessons were showing progress and I was understanding the importance of music on our mental wellbeing, I was thinking more about sounds, and effects they can have on our feelings. I thought about the music tape that the clinic I had taken him to as a young child had given me to play several times a day to help with his sensitive hearing. I saw how it had a calming effect upon him. Now, all these years later he was enjoying singing and playing the keyboard, which was a miracle I never thought possible!

The effects it was having on Jonathan and other members made me realise that there was a connection to music, and the beneficial outcomes it could have upon my autistic son. I wanted to learn more about it.

I had new ideas on how to help our members to encourage eye contact. Autistic people find it very difficult to look at someone. Although I continued to help members to make eye contact as much as possible. I understood how difficult it was for them at times, and continual encouragement and motivation helped to build their confidence over time.

In the music group some members would look down or turn to the side rather than look at other people in the group. The idea I had for the new year was to purchase a monitor and camera so they could look at themselves on the screen and therefore not be anxious about others looking at them. It could also encourage eye contact just seeing their own face on the screen. I felt that it was an opportunity I had to try. Another idea I wanted to introduce in our music group was self-expression through movement. I could encourage and involve the members together. Jonathan liked songs about trains and my intention was to get him to do train movements or sounds if certain songs had words which we could express with our hands, like smiling, or sad, or love. I felt it would be a wonderful way of helping those who were less verbal to express themselves in their own way. They could make their own props to help them. It would connect the creative art group to the music group by painting or drawing whatever picture helped them with their song. I had a strong feeling that the idea would help Jonathan and the others to expand upon their progress in confidence. Facial expression and movements would help with their coordination too.

Jonathan did not understand acting, or drama; his autism meant that his imagination does not enable him to 'pretend', or role play. He can only relate to that which he sees. Even as a child imaginary play was not part of his development as it is with children who are not autistic. Encouraging expression through music and being able to see how they look and move is like acting in a different way that suits their needs.

Having devoted my life to helping my son, trying to understand about how his autism affects his life, I have struggled through many difficult years to give my son as many opportunities as I could that would help him progress in any way, however small or more than I had expected. I always believed in his ability to learn, and if he is encouraged and given opportunities he will continue to develop.

I reached the depths of despair many times because I could not see him ever improving. His behaviour was getting more challenging and difficult at times for me to cope with. I felt a complete failure as a mother, with no support. I had to keep finding the strength and determination to go on. It was little steps of progress when I least expected any that kept me going, because it was proving that my son had the ability to learn.

Jonathan has grown into a loving, caring adult who is continuing to progress in ways I thought impossible, however much I had hoped! His wood carving skills are quite amazing, as are his keyboard skills, and all the other activities he had done well at like archery, table tennis, bowling, train driving. He has raised awareness of autism and the capabilities autistic people have. I feel society has a long way to go yet in understanding autism.

All the issues I have been working on with Jonathan over the years are ongoing, but looking at him now, I feel and realise his progress had advanced after all the difficulties he had as a young child. When the private clinic explained the reasons for his behaviour, and reactions to sound, different textures, his dislike of clothes, foods and smells, it all made sense to me.

I knew if I did not work on those problems, the fear of him being institutionalised could come true. His behaviour was so challenging and I wasn't sure how long I would be able to cope with him. Having these explanations for his behaviour, with a programme of things to do which may help him, gave me some hope of being able to help him. I had to try, even though I didn't know if he had any future or quality of life.

I felt excited about starting another year of developing our creative art and music, as I had new ideas to introduce to help Jonathan and the other members to progress. I purchased a monitor and camera with the aim of encouraging the members to make eye contact with each other. It was a difficult concept to begin with as the members did not like looking at themselves on the screen, or 'television' as they related to it as. Jonathan did not like looking at photographs of himself and did not want any on display at home. I felt and hoped that the camera, and being able to see himself sing, dance and use actions to his songs may build his confidence over time and help the other members. When he was growing up, he was not interested in looking at photographs of himself. I realised that it was connected to his autism, and I hadn't found a way to work on that issue until the idea came to me as I was developing the group.

As members gradually got used to seeing themselves on 'television' (as they liked to call it) they were starting to enjoy it! I could see the improvements in Jonathan showing emotion when singing and making facial expressions. This was amazing progress for him, because he was putting his own feelings across. This I knew was wonderful progress in his development. I had learnt over the years that his autism made it extremely difficult for him to express feelings other than becoming stressed, anxious or loud. When singing, he was relating to the words. If they were words that described happy or sad feelings, his tone of voice and facial expressions would change to express those emotions. I knew that I had found another way of helping him to express himself through music and the positive outcomes that could be built on. Jonathan and the other members were proving they could achieve if given the opportunity!

Both the music and creative art groups were developing in the way I had hoped and aimed for. I took the camera and monitor into the creative art group every few weeks to encourage the members to show their art on camera and say a few words about it, again encouraging eye contact and communication skills.

They all enjoyed being on 'television'. Jonathan continued to progress in keyboard skills and wood carving. I was always looking for new experiences for him to try. I came across a leaflet posted in a local shop for pottery classes. It was local, so I took the details to find out more. I felt that Jonathan had shown skills in wood carving; maybe pottery might be something he would like. Not knowing anything about pottery, I phoned to ask what the costs were, and if Jonathan could join the group with me supporting him. To my surprise, the person who was teaching pottery was very happy for Jonathan to go along and try. She assured me that he would be made welcome, and informed me that she had experience of working with autistic people! After talking about it to Jonathan we decided to go and look at the small group. They made us feel very welcome, and the person teaching showed Jonathan all the different things she had made. He was interested in looking at the clay, the potter's wheel, and watching a demonstration on how to use it. Jonathan was happy about going back, when he could wear his clothes to 'work' in (as he didn't like getting dirty). I explained to the person teaching that he would have to wear his 'working' clothes and shoes before trying pottery; I wasn't sure if he would like getting his hands full of clay, but it was a wonderful opportunity for him to try.

We joined the group the following week. With the wood carving group, every beginner had made a leaf. As it was pottery, everyone made a bowl. Jonathan was shown how to use the clay and form it into a bowl. I was observing Jonathan, looking at the way he was using his hands to gently form a bowl shape. It took quite a while. He was concentrating on trying to get the shape of a bowl right! He didn't seem to worry how much clay he had on his hands. This, I thought, was wonderful progress for his dexterity and sensory issues skills. Feeling the texture of the clay and moulding it was amazing to see.

Again, working on the sensory issues over the years was proving to be beneficial. I was so pleased about this. I knew he would like doing pottery as it was a small group and a calm environment where Jonathan was accepted and encouraged by the other members. They were very talented at pottery!

Again, trying to raise awareness of autism, I encouraged Jonathan to talk about the wood carving group and creative art and music groups to help others, who may not have had any contact or experience with autistic people, to understand that Jonathan and others did have the ability to learn and achieve, if they were given the opportunity.

The pottery group was going very well. Jonathan was enjoying it and learning very quickly. The person who was teaching felt that Jonathan was now ready to try the potter's wheel. I understood that it would be difficult at first to control the clay and wheel. When I watched Jonathan with his first attempt at doing the wheel, I expected the clay to go everywhere. I was absolutely amazed at the coordination and control he demonstrated when using the potter's wheel. The teacher was so pleased at the skill Jonathan was showing. She had not experienced any of the students being able to control the wheel as well as Jonathan had shown. I was so happy! My son was proving that he could learn new skills.

By giving him as many opportunities as possible, he was developing different skills. He continued to amaze me, and the label of 'autistic' was not going to stop him proving his capabilities.

Over time, Jonathan went on to make some wonderful pottery items. One object was a train, which he enjoyed making very much. It did take a number of weeks, as each part of the train had to dry out before the next stage could begin. Jonathan understood about the waiting time for clay to dry; this was a learning experience too. With wood carving he could complete an object quickly, but pottery was different. I was so pleased that he had the opportunity with the pottery group, but I felt that he would soon reach a stage where he had learnt and enjoyed all he wanted to. He had made some lovely dishes, bowls, jugs, and trains which he had painted at the pottery classes (they needed special paints). He had reached the stage of wanting to finish at that group. I explained to the teacher that he had no further interest in the pottery class. The teacher understood completely, and was so pleased to have had Jonathan in the group. I felt that Jonathan was happy continuing his wood carving group and the creative art and music group. I felt pleased that he had the opportunity and brought it to a natural end himself. It helped me realise what was important to Jonathan: he was choosing the things that he wanted to do! It was what I had been working towards over all the long years.

I was continuing to learn about my son's autism and how it affected him. Seeing just how his skills developed in wood carving and pottery was wonderful.

He had made objects that he could relate to, like a train, bowl, leaves or jugs. He did not have an imagination to create something different. It had to be things which he could see and were 'real' to him. As a child, imaginary play was difficult for him. I felt that it was part of his autism. In our creative art group, he would draw or paint trains, boats or things he had seen, or places he had visited, like castles or railway stations. Although I would try and encourage him to do something different, he would always go back to that which he could relate to. In the music group, he enjoyed singing a wide range of songs and seeing himself on the monitor. I could see the progress it was having on Jonathan's confidence, his expression and his communication skills.

Encouraging expression through actions was enjoyable for him and the other members. I could see how Jonathan was using more facial expressions because he could see himself on the screen. He was becoming more aware of the feelings he was trying to express, and how he looked when putting those emotions into his songs. It was wonderful to see his progress and realise we had found something that will continue to build his confidence. Having a safe and happy environment to socialise and express himself is important to his progress.

Of all of the activities Jonathan has had the opportunity to experience, he feels settled and happy with the art and music group, which is having amazing positive outcomes on his development. His communication skills are continuing to improve, as is his confidence. His keyboard lessons and the ability to understand musical notes is amazing. Chris, his teacher, is finding ways in which to help Jonathan develop and expand upon the pieces of music he can play, as well as the variety. My hope is that Jonathan will one day be able to play some classical music. Chris has assured me that Jonathan has the ability to achieve that.

My son is approaching twenty-five years old. It has taken many years of struggling, hardship, emotional and physical exhaustion to keep going. It is the love and belief I have in my son that motivated me and made me determined to give him a life with quality that he deserves. I would not give up on him and 'find a home to put him in' as I was advised to do with him when he was a child. I did not understand autism, but I devoted my life to trying to help my son cope with the devasting effects being autistic can have on your child's life, and family.

In our case, one consequence was the breakdown of the family unit, when one parent found it too difficult to accept the diagnosis of their child being autistic. My daughter decided to disown me because she could not understand my drive to help her brother, whom she and her father considered not worthwhile. It has been many years now since any contact had taken place with my son's father or his sibling. They have not seen the progress as I have of Jonathan achieving so much in so many ways. It saddens me that they rejected him and blamed me for the decisions I made to help my son as much as possible, rather than to 'find a home to put him in'.

Jonathan has grown into a loving, caring person. He displays empathy towards the members of our art and music group. If anyone is upset about something, he will go to them to ask if they are alright or take a tissue if they are crying.

These spontaneous reactions are very moving to see, and show just how the friendships and respect for each other have developed. This has proven that the groups were the right environment to nurture those emotions and it's wonderful to see!

Our kind and caring volunteer, John, who has supported me and my vision for Uniquely Me & U, wrote a motto which describes what our group stands for, and describes it perfectly in a few words: Love us, respect us, in us believe, given opportunity we will achieve.

Those words are so meaningful and describe how I have cared for my son over his life. By forming the groups and helping others with autism and learning disabilities to socialise and develop their talents, and to feel part of the community.

Jonathan is enjoying the music group and still progressing. He is expanding his choice of songs and writing out the lyrics to type them onto the computer to print out to keep in his folders. He likes looking at himself on the screen and his emotional expressive actions are becoming more meaningful, which is so encouraging to see. His keyboard skills are amazing, and I am so proud of how far he has come in his development. I can honestly say that I feel truly happy for him. For myself, his mother, who had no idea that, through all the different opportunities I would give Jonathan, it would be music and playing a keyboard that was going to have such amazing, wonderful, outcomes on his continued progress.

The clinic I took him to as a young child explained his sensitive hearing and how different sounds affected him. I am exploring a therapy called Harmonic Sound Healing, with the tape that the clinic had suggested I played to help Jonathan for his sensitive hearing when he was a child. I saw the calming effects it had on him then. Learning about sounds and notes on a keyboard or piano makes a great deal of sense to me, and how it could help me to further understand Jonathan's choice in music, and his autism in relation to music.

Through the experience of devoting my life to caring for my son and trying to understand how autism affected him, there was always something different to learn about his complex issues. Music and sound provide other opportunities to learn about and help my son.

Over the years I have tried to deal with every issue which my son had difficulties with and tried to find ways to overcome and manage them on a daily basis. With no help or support, or professional guidance, I have had to deal with these impossible issues alone. This took me to the limits of my emotional and physical capabilities, but each glimpse of progress that my son made helped me to keep going. I believed that Jonathan had the ability to learn, and I as his mother (and all he had) needed to focus on that, which I did.

My son is continuing to progress, and is a caring, loving person. Our lives are more peaceful, meaningful, and I now enjoy the person Jonathan has become. I no longer dread each day, and the difficult problems which a challenging autistic child, with what seems little hope of improving, can have.

My journey has been extremely challenging, but worthwhile. I hope it may help others who are caring for an autistic person to nurture the skills that person has, and to respect the fact that we are all different and learn in different ways.

The word 'normal' and its expectations can be as challenging as the label 'autistic'. We need to understand everyone as individuals, and to accept everyone as individuals; we all have a right to be included within a caring society, to be cared for, and be listened to.

Acknowledgements

I would like to thank

Mike Watkins - for giving up his time voluntary at the heritage railway, to help Jonathan develop his interest in trains. Giving him the opportunity to gain a variety of skills using different tools, which has proved invaluable over the years.

Alan Payne FGNI MAHM consultant Herbalist and Naturopathic Iridologist – for his continued help with Jonathan's physical and emotional wellbeing. Which has had beneficial outcomes, and enabled him to cope with many issues his autism has brought out.

Michael Painter – A.R.B.S Royal Society of Sculptors – for giving Jonathan the opportunity to try wood carving, and discovering he has the ability to learn other skills.

Chris Watts – keyboard and piano teacher, who has encouraged Jonathan to develop his ability to play the keyboard, read music, and he is continuing to progress in his musical skills.

John Philips – for his voluntary support with the music and creative art groups.

Rachael Tierney – for her help and skills.

ABS computers, Mark and Simon for their technical support.

Tina Tarrant – for her art work.

Julie Barratt – Harmonic Sound Healing therapist – for introducing a therapy about how different sounds can have beneficial effects on our mental wellbeing.